STRATEGIC WEIGHT LOSS

STRATEGIC WEIGHT LOSS

20 Practical and Effective Strategies for Lifelong Success

By Cynthia Clarke, RN, BSN, MA

Surrogate Press®

Published in the United States by
Surrogate Press®
an imprint of Faceted Press®
Surrogate Press, LLC
Park City, Utah
SurrogatePress.com

ISBN: 978-1-947459-99-1
Library of Congress Control Number: 2024906609

Book cover design by: Michelle Rayner, Cosmic Design LLC
Interior design by: Katie Mullaly, Surrogate Press®

Terms of Use

Strategic Weight Loss is written and published as an information resource and educational guide for both professionals and non-professionals. It should not be used as a substitute for your physician's advice. Be sure to work with a physician who knows the importance of diet in healing and wellbeing. While the author endorses *Strategic Weight Loss* and related recommendations, you should make your decisions based on all the information at hand, knowing that you are the primary force in directing your own life and health.

Table of Contents

Preface

About this book and how to use it...

This book is the culmination of over thirty years' worth of experiential learning, trial and error practices, and formal nutrition study. Additionally, I have a Bachelor of Science in Dietetics and Nutrition as well as a Bachelor of Science in Nursing. I worked directly with clients as both a nutrition counselor and personal trainer.

Mostly, though, these strategies have been formulated through my personal experience struggling with my own weight problem as a child and young adult. What resulted was a passionate quest to constantly strive to improve my fitness and healthy lifestyle.

This book and the strategies within it are grouped by dietary, movement/exercise, and mindset strategies. I personally find it easier to use a systematic approach, and I felt it was necessary to organize the strategies by relative groupings. However, they do not necessarily need to be read in order. The book can—and should—be used according to what works best for you. If it feels easier or makes more sense to start with the mindset strategies, or to move around from chapter to chapter, each strategy can stand on its own whether you read the chapters consecutively or not, with the exception of The Preparation and The Introduction, which should be read first.

The most important goal for each chapter is to read it thoroughly and then practice the strategy until it is fully incorporated into your daily habits before moving on to the next.

PART I
Introduction

Introduction to Strategic Weight Loss

Why strategies? What does that mean, exactly? Why not a diet plan?

When I was a young kid, I learned very quickly through constant teasing and bullying that there was something different about me. I didn't look like the other kids around me at school. I was really overweight, and all the other kids seemed to be skinny and petite. The bullies reminded me of that every day. It got so bad that my own sister wouldn't let me sit next to her on the school bus, I imagine, for fear of association.

But the weight wasn't just affecting how I looked. In gym class, I had a decidedly slower pace on the track, a sort of clumsiness in my movements, and a definite lack of energy compared to my schoolmates. Most of the other kids looked forward to heading outside for gym class. I wanted to go hide in a bathroom stall.

It was a horrible time in my life. The constant bullying led to depression and suicidal thoughts. I had trouble making friends and my self-esteem was under constant assault. I was desperate for relief and searched relentlessly for solutions. My circumstances took a heavy toll on my young mind. However, in retrospect, it was the beginning of what eventually led me to a rewarding lifelong journey pursuing health and fitness.

Starting from a young age, I tried everything from weight loss meetings with embarrassing weigh-ins to every conceivable diet plan, diet pill, and supplement. I also experimented with multiple types of exercise. I began running, biking, and taking aerobics classes whenever I could.

Through all my efforts and each new approach, I finally came to a profound conclusion. My eventual success with weight loss didn't have anything to do with any particular diet plan or specific exercise. It all boiled down to the strategies I was naturally developing over time throughout the totality of my experience. For example, I discovered early on that I was totally compliant in sticking to exercise *only* if I got it done in the morning. If I waited until the afternoon, I would lose my motivation. Planning morning workouts has been a mainstay in my schedule ever since.

Another strategy I developed came by way of accepting that I have a big sweet tooth. Life got a lot easier when I stopped trying to force myself into various "sugar-free challenges." That approach backfired on me every single time! Now I keep reasonably healthy sweets on hand so I can satisfy cravings without going off the deep end. I've also learned through working with clients that if there's something in their daily diet that they cannot live without, I don't try and convince them to give it up. That only causes panic and resistance. Coffee is a perfect example. Morning coffee is a *ritual* for many people. I would never try and take that away. Instead, I might offer alternatives to the heavy doses of cream and sugar they have been adding and give them time to adapt.

The strategies I cultivated are simple, practical, daily habits that naturally lead to healthy lifestyle changes. They not only improved my health, but they also improved my relationship with food and exercise.

How to Work Through The Strategies

I believe the best way to approach the strategies laid out in this book is to focus on one strategy at a time. Read through each strategy and highlight the helpful tips as you go. Place your attention on developing new habits and behavior modifications before you move forward.

Choose the right pace for yourself to experience small successes and build the momentum you need to continue progressing. Small, *healthy* habits cultivated over time yield big results. If you find that you need to focus on a particular strategy longer than the others, I encourage you to follow your instinct and take the time you need before moving on. There is no need to rush. The most important thing to remember is that you are creating new habits that put you on a trajectory toward a healthier way of living. It's normal to crave fast results, but if you become overwhelmed, you are more likely to fall back into bad habits.

You might want to dog-ear some of the tougher strategies to revisit later, after you've made progress with the ones that feel easier. It's important to have some wins as you move forward and to not fall back into a defeatist mindset.

A FINAL NOTE ON DIETS

Every couple of years a new type of diet phenomenon takes hold and grabs tons of media attention. I've seen my share of diets and diet products come and go. Some have lived on longer than they should. I make no claims here about any specific diet. These strategies are applicable to virtually any diet plan. The strategies have more to do with habits of daily living that lead to overall success. However, if you plan to simultaneously try the strategies along with a diet plan, whether it is Keto, Paleo, a diabetic plan, etc., the most important thing is that it is nutritionally balanced.

It is your choice, but I would like to emphasize that the strategies will work with *almost* any style of eating or "diet." My hope is that whatever plan you try, you continue to apply these strategies. As a result, you'll discover that true freedom from your weight loss struggles can last a lifetime.

The Preparation

Failing to prepare is preparing to fail.
Benjamin Franklin

You must understand that losing weight and maintaining it does not come from a "diet." It doesn't come from any type of temporary restriction you complete after a period of time. There is also no magic in any diet or supplement. Long-term-weight-loss success and health comes from making sustainable lifestyle changes. It comes from small changes you make every day and the simple habits you stick with consistently over time.

Preparing for a new lifestyle simply requires a willingness to recognize that you are not defective because you've struggled to lose or maintain your weight. You've just collected a group of habits that don't support your positive intention. The great news is that the right strategies can empower anyone to build a foundation for lasting success.

Before jumping into the strategies, however, I must cover some of the basics of the physiology of how weight gain and weight loss works. I don't care what anyone tells you or what you've read. I don't care what diets you've tried in the past or what any "health guru" proclaims. There is one basic rule of body weight and it's purely scientific whether you like this rule or not. It does not change from diet to diet.

The Rule: To lose weight, the body must burn more calories than it consumes.

This principle refers to a "caloric deficit." Any self-described expert that tells you otherwise is not only lying and denying basic physiology, but they are more than likely trying to sell you something. You might find success using an approach like intermittent fasting, the Keto diet, the Paleo diet, etc., but the magic isn't in the food. It's usually the fact that there's something about that style of eating that has you eating fewer calories than you were prior to starting. There's nothing wrong with that. If something is working for you and it's nutritionally balanced, then go for it! But it's important that you're clear about *why* it's working.

Here are some other facts:

We can physiologically only lose about one percent of our total body weight per week (or approximately up to two pounds). Additional losses are most often water fluctuations.

It takes *approximately* a 3,500-calorie deficit to lose one pound of body fat[1].

While I don't personally love math, I can assure you that getting familiar with a few simple equations along with some basic principles of physiology will serve you well in the long run. It's understandable why weight loss can be so challenging for most people when you need to find a few thousand calories to cut out for every pound you want to lose. Don't despair…this is where the strategies come in. It is possible. This leads us to a few easy preparation tasks I want you to complete before moving forward.

---

1 The 3,500-calorie deficit is impacted by multiple variables. It is used for general reference only.

TASK ONE

Get a new notebook (or an electronic version) to record your progress and keep track of some basic information. On the first few pages, I want you to write down the equations that follow. These include a few simple calculations that will come in handy and help you establish a starting point for yourself. These calculations are *guidelines only*. The numbers you get provide you with a reference point from which to start. This is important because if you know what your baseline is, then you can accurately track your progress and adjust where needed.

The Body Mass Index Formula (also referred to as BMI)

The first of the two calculations is the body mass index (BMI) formula, which is often used by medical professionals as a rudimentary measurement of health. Its aim is to provide a *general* picture of your body fat based on your height and weight. There are obvious limitations to this calculation. **It cannot possibly account for variations in body composition**. The only truly accurate way to measure body fat is using hydrostatic underwater weighing, which is typically done at universities that have specialized equipment and full-body Dexa scan. Dexa scan measures several components of body composition in addition to body fat percentage including bone density and lean muscle tissue. If you don't have access to either of those, this equation gives an *approximation* of body fat to total mass. It may be useful in tracking progress.

BMI is used by most healthcare professionals, so it gives you another tool for communicating with your physician if they want to discuss your weight.

(Weight in pounds ÷ (Height in inches x Height in inches)) x 703

Use a calculator or use one of the ready-made calculators online, which are much easier. There are several websites that have an easy calculator where you just plug in your height and weight. A quick search will pull up several options. When you get your BMI number, use it to compare it to the BMI categories as follows:

Underweight: <18.5
Normal Weight: 18.5–24.9
Overweight: 25–29.9
Obese: 30 or greater

The BMR Formula

The next calculation is Basal Metabolic Rate or BMR. This is an estimation of the number of calories your body burns at rest over a twenty-four-hour period. *This does not account for activity.*

Women: 65.5 + (4.35 x weight in pounds) + (4.7 x height in inches) – (4.7 x age in years)

Men: 66 + (6.23 x weight in pounds) + (12.7 x height in inches) – (6.8 x age in years)

Again, search for an online calculator to make this easier. Record the number you get in your notebook. Your BMR is important to know because it gives you a baseline of calories required for weight maintenance. It is worth noting that there are clinics that offer a simple test to determine BMR which uses a calorimeter device you breathe into. Check your area for availability. The next equation will factor in activity.

The Harris Benedict Equation

This equation helps you determine *approximately*, based on your average activity level, how many calories you likely burn on a given day. You need to take an honest assessment of your true activity level while understanding that your activity levels often fluctuate from day to day. Choose the activity level closest to a *typical* day. You will need the number you calculated for your BMR.

Sedentary (little to no exercise): BMR x 1.2

Light Activity (light exercise 1–3 days per week): BMR x 1.375

Moderate Activity (moderate exercise 3–4 days per week): BMR x 1.55

Very Active (hard exercise 6–7 days per week): BMR x 1.725

Extra Active (very hard sports and/or physical job): BMR x 1.9

This is not an exact science, of course. But it's a starting point in determining *roughly* how many calories your body needs just to maintain your current weight. The following is an example using all the equations together, so you get a complete picture of how to use these numbers as a tool for weight loss:

Take, for example, a thirty-five-year-old female who is 5'5" and 165 lbs. and does light exercise on a weekly basis. Using the calculations above, we can determine that her BMI is 27.5, which puts her in the "overweight" category. Based on her age, her BMR is 1,610 calories per day. Adjusting for her light activity, her baseline calories would be around 2,214 calories per day for weight *maintenance.*

Of course, this is all an estimation, but the way we know for sure how many calories she needs to maintain her weight is to start tracking her daily calories. If her weight stayed the same after a couple of weeks while eating roughly 2,200 calories per day, as her BMR suggests, then that would be an indication that the calculations were correct. From that point, we would know that if she wanted to lose weight, she would need to decrease some of her daily calories (as well as increase activity).

If this all seems like too much work, I get it. This is why fad diets are so attractive. They are designed to make us believe that we'll never have to do any work if we just follow *their* program. This way does take extra thought and it does take extra work in the beginning, but this approach empowers you with the fundamental knowledge you need to turn small habits—combined with a little work—into lasting results. And I promise you it gets easier with time, patience, and consistency.

TASK TWO

I strongly encourage you to make an appointment with your healthcare provider for an annual check-up. Not only is it an excellent practice to have an annual check-up, but it also gives you a baseline of your current state of health. Bring your notebook with you (unless you have an online portal where you can access all your appointment notes) and keep a record of your vital signs, lab results, etc. That way, when you go back a year later, you can compare. It's genuinely gratifying to see labs and vital signs improve after you've been putting in the effort. Those are markers many of us never pay attention to, yet they will reflect your good habits and provide more positive feedback to reinforce your *new* habits. Plus, you'll have peace of mind knowing that you're taking care of your health.

TASK THREE

The final task to complete before moving ahead is to clean out your refrigerator and pantry. Clean and organize the shelves and throw out or donate any foods that you know are unhealthy and feel ready to let go of (think chips, candy, etc.). As you go through the strategies, there will be changes you naturally make along the way, but to set a positive tone and make your intentions official, it's important to start fresh with a supportive environment. The simple act of organizing and preparing will help you create a healthier relationship with your kitchen environment.

Set aside a few hours to complete this task. It's important that you take the time to organize everything for easy access. You want to be able to see the foods you have and to make sure anything that is expired is thrown out. Reading labels and understanding what you choose to eat is part of this process. It's also part of educating yourself to make better choices in the future.

Two of my top guidelines for reading labels:

1. Ingredients are listed in the order of quantity used in making the product. That means if sugar is the first listed ingredient, then the label is telling you there is more sugar in that product than any other ingredient listed. That's something to avoid! It doesn't matter if the sweetness comes from white sugar, refined sugar, molasses, honey, or high fructose syrup. Those are all variations of sugar, and you want to avoid products that have it listed as the first three or four ingredients.
2. Look at the number of calories per serving. Then, look at the *number of servings* in one package! I emphasize this because you can buy a packaged cookie, for example, and discover that one cookie is listed as two servings. This is manufacturing trickery! It's a very common dupe and they hope you won't notice, but you *will* notice now and understand exactly what you're getting inside that package.

Please don't skip this very important task. I'm a big believer, through my own experience, that making the effort to clear and prepare your space has a direct impact on the probability of success. It gets you ready mentally and emotionally for the changes you'll make along the way.

PART II
Nourishment Strategies
Food / Diet

STRATEGY 1
Liquid Calories

"I can't change the direction of the wind,
but I can adjust my sails to always reach my destination."
Jimmy Dean

This is my number one strategy to get healthier and drop excess weight. It can be your single most effective tool depending on how much soda, juice, or energy drinks you currently consume on a daily basis.

The average American drinks forty-two gallons of sugary beverages per year, which is the equivalent to thirty-nine pounds of sugar. And the problem is not just added sugar; it's also what is lacking. Consider this: if you compare eating an orange versus drinking a glass of orange juice, you can see why you should always *eat* your calories rather than *drink* them.

A 6-ounce glass of orange juice, unsweetened has:

339 calories, 81 total carbohydrates, 79.8 grams of sugar, and 1.7 grams of fiber.

A raw navel orange has:

69 calories, 17 total carbohydrates, 11.9 grams of sugar, and 3.1 grams of fiber.

So, not only will it be more satisfying to eat a whole orange because solid foods are more filling, but the difference in calories is staggering! Eating the whole orange has significantly fewer calories, less grams of sugar, and (bonus!) more fiber. Fiber fills you up and helps you feel satisfied longer, so more fiber equals greater satiety.

Drinking your calories is a guaranteed diet destroyer. It's the same with electrolyte and energy drinks. Electrolyte drinks are deceptively marketed as health and athletic performance enhancers, which tricks you into thinking they are good for you. Look at the label. Most of those drinks are loaded with sugar and calories. You must eliminate these drinks if you want to live a healthy lifestyle.

For example, I had a male client who was very active in outdoor sports. Despite his intense activity levels, he struggled with his weight and had some joint pain. He told me he was trying to eat healthy but couldn't figure out why the weight wouldn't budge. We talked about what a typical day of eating looked like for him, and his choices seemed reasonable. So, I dug a little deeper and I asked him to tell me *everything* he was drinking throughout the day.

This client started his day with a glass of orange juice, then typically drank a couple cans of soda with his meals, and often ended his day with a glass of milk with his dessert or a snack. The average calories in a can of soda is about 150 calories. Add in the juice and milk and he was getting an extra 560 calories per day in drinks alone. Over the course of one week, that would total 3,920 calories.

Once I showed him the math, he felt motivated to give up the daily sodas and orange juice. But he really enjoyed his nightly milk. So, I swapped out his whole milk for unsweetened almond milk. To his surprise, he preferred the almond milk and adapted quickly to the new taste.

This client ended up losing forty pounds over the course of one year, primarily focusing on liquid calories and not much else! Losing the extra weight seemed to alleviate a good deal of his joint pain, too. He was amazed with the success he had simply by eliminating liquid calories. I've spoken with him many times since, and he always comments on how easily he lost weight with such small changes.

If you are drinking calories, this will be the most dramatic change you make all year. I encourage you to focus solely on this strategy until you have eliminated all sugar-filled drinks before moving on. This is challenging, but when you embrace this strategy, your body will be much better off for it. A diet high in sugar has been associated with a greater risk of Type 2 Diabetes, certain cancers, and an increased risk of dying from heart disease.

The key is to make this transition sustainable. Growing up, I was addicted to soda. I drank several cans and fountain drinks every day. Switching to diet soda didn't help me kick my habit. In my many attempts going cold turkey, I realized I needed a substitute. I discovered that sparkling water was satisfying in place of soda. It was the strategy that worked for me, and I don't miss the soda at all.

Coffee-Shop Drinks

I can't talk about liquid calories without addressing coffee, chai, or other coffee-shop drinks. The actual coffee or tea is not the problem. But all the junk that goes into it can turn your coffee into a liquid dessert. If you are someone who likes to go to your local coffee shop and order something decadent each day, this will be a major wake-up call because the ones that have a lot of cream, syrups, and whipped cream added are shockingly high in calories. Just glancing at one major coffee chain's nutrition content, I found coffee drinks that were 420 calories (and up to 570 calories in the larger size). That's a staggering number of calories for one drink! But you don't need to give it all up and drink your coffee black. I do have modifications to suggest, though.

For example, if you're not ready to give up your favorite drink, try a smaller size and have it made with sugar-free syrup. Leave the whipped cream off. Another option is to look at the nutrition menu, find out the calories in your current order, and browse through the menu to find a similar option that has at least one hundred fewer calories.

This is how you make lasting changes. You don't need to be ultra strict and feel deprived every day. The lasting changes are the ones that are sustainable for you. When it comes to coffee, maybe you *are* someone who can easily decide to stop going out and make it at home. Maybe that doesn't work for you. That's okay, too. Be realistic about what you can reasonably achieve. That's why this book is about strategies…not a particular diet plan that rigidly makes certain foods "bad" and other foods "good."

This applies to tea drinkers, as well as any other special drink you regularly have. Look at what's in your tea, matcha, chai, etc. Is it cream and sugar? Are you pouring a bottle of honey into your drink? Honey and sugar are not "bad," but you must start measuring the amount of your add-ins and look up the calories. Then, adjust the quantity or replace it with something better. If you realize you've been using one-third cup of cream each day, reduce that to just two to three tablespoons.

Also consider that coffees and teas are stimulating. They make us feel alert. I recommend not consuming any caffeine after 3:00 pm. Even *that* might be too late in the day for you. We all metabolize caffeine differently and some are more sensitive to it than others. Drinking coffee or tea late in the day can affect your sleep and it makes some people feel jittery or anxious. If you have these issues, decrease the amount of coffee you drink or make sure you cut yourself off earlier and earlier until you are no longer having sleep disruptions.

On the positive side, caffeine is a performance enhancer. Research shows that when people have a moderate amount of caffeine prior to a work-out, they work out harder and make a greater effort. Additional research suggests that coffee drinking, within healthy limits, *may* have protective benefits against Parkinson's disease and Type 2 Diabetes and a decreased risk of depression.

Coffee and tea are not problematic from a weight loss perspective, but what you add to it makes a huge difference. Take the time to evaluate either the nutrition menu at your favorite coffee spot or the ingredients you add to your drinks at home.

When you eliminate sodas and juices, it is also important to replace the unhealthy habit with one that is beneficial. Drinking adequate water is important for good health and staying hydrated helps with appetite control and energy levels.

Practical Strategies for ELIMINATING LIQUID CALORIES

1. Phase in Water.
2. Drink your first liter of water before you leave the house in the morning to get a head start.
3. Buy a reusable water bottle and fill it up throughout the day.
4. Keep a fresh batch of herbal iced tea ready in the refrigerator so you always have a non-caffeinated option.

5. Keep sparkling mineral water in your kitchen at home and at work as an alternative to soda.
6. Pick up a few different brands of calorie-free drink flavorings like Mio or Crystal Light. They come in several different flavors that you add to your water. These types of products can help a lot when you are used to drinking soda throughout the day.
7. If you and your kids drink orange juice at breakfast, swap regular juice for a low-sugar version or start by mixing the low-sugar version with the regular orange juice (a half and half mix) and gradually switch entirely to the low-sugar O.J. Your kids are much less likely to notice the swap if you do it gradually and without mentioning it or making a big deal about it.

Practical Strategies for Coffee-Shop Drinks:

1. Look up the drink you currently order. Ask: *How many calories are in my favorite drink?*
2. Be aware of what you consume. Ask: *Can I make a small change today?*
3. Look at the size of your drink. Ask: *Can I get something smaller?*
4. Look at the ingredients. Ask: *Can I swap out any of the ingredients for lower-calorie versions (sugar-free syrup, low-fat milk instead of full-fat, almond milk instead of full-fat milk or cream)?*
5. Look at the toppings. Ask: *Can I order without whipped cream and syrup on top?*

AT HOME:

1. Review your coffee/tea ritual. Ask: *What am I putting into my drinks and what is the nutrition content/calories and fat?*
2. Look at the amount of coffee/tea you have throughout the day. Ask: *Can I cut down by a small degree (maybe have one less cup than usual)?*
3. Look at what you add to your drinks. Ask: *Am I willing to measure my cream/sugar?* If I just dump in cream, for example, am I willing to measure it and possibly reduce the amount?

OTHER STRATEGIES:

1. Try Stevia or monk fruit/lakanto as natural sweeteners, or other natural sweeteners that have zero calories.
2. Use non-dairy creamers (coconut or almond milk creamer), which tend to be lower in fat and calories than half and half.
3. Measure what you consume using a measuring cup or tablespoons. Know what you're drinking and how much. Condition yourself to be aware of what you eat and drink each day. Learn what true portion sizes look like.

STRATEGY 2

The Breakfast Strategy

With the new day comes new strength and new thoughts.

Eleanor Roosevelt

Most trainers and fitness experts agree that it's important to start your day with a good meal. Breakfast can kick-start your energy and it helps prevent bingeing and poor food choices later in the morning. There are also studies that link a pattern of skipping breakfast with an increased risk of obesity.

One study compared subjects given the same number of calories each day. One group split their calories between lunch and dinner (skipping breakfast) while the other group split their calories across breakfast, lunch, and dinner. The group that included the breakfast meal lost more weight than the other group at the end of the trial.

Having a healthy meal in the morning also sets you on a positive trajectory for the day. When you have a routine planned and you stick with it, it will influence your state of mind.

Plan your morning the night before. Set your alarm and allow time for breakfast. Decide what you're going to eat in advance so you can make a thoughtful choice. The more smoothly your morning goes, the more likely you are to start your day with a positive attitude. Don't allow your first meal to be an afterthought or a lazy habit that you repeat over and over without any consideration.

A friend of mine once asked me to help him out with his diet. He was a man in his early forties who lived a mostly sedentary life except for the occasional golf game. He didn't have an obvious *weight* problem of any kind, but he knew he wanted to get healthier. He just didn't feel like he was at his best, physically.

This was someone who was fortunate enough to take an early retirement and he happened to be single without any kids or pets. So, his lifestyle didn't necessitate a strict schedule of any kind. He was able to wake up when he wanted with no pressing obligations.

I asked him to tell me about his morning routine and what he ate for breakfast. I often like to look at a client's breakfast and their morning routine first because I know that if you can master your morning, the rest of the day will flow much better. It's also more effective to work on changing one or two habits at a time.

He told me that he typically slept in and, after getting out of bed, he'd throw on some clothes and go to the local donut shop drive-through. His usual order consisted of two donuts plus a large coffee with cream and sugar.

The first thing I asked him to do was to start setting his alarm to establish a consistent wake pattern. Regular sleep/wake times are important for restful sleep, but I also wanted him to return structure to his day. The next step was making some adjustments to his breakfast. I didn't want to take away his donut shop routine because it was something he enjoyed, but we talked about healthier alternatives and adjustments he could make. For example, I asked him to choose either a smaller sized coffee *or* swap milk in place of the half and half in his large coffee.

The next change he agreed to make was to order an egg sandwich they offered in lieu of the donuts. It was a healthier choice we could both live with. The protein in the egg sandwich would keep him satisfied longer and it drastically reduced the amount of sugar he ate.

The small changes he made in his morning routine led to healthier choices throughout the day because he felt proud that he was able to stick with his new plan. The consistent wake time meant that he had to go to bed earlier, and the regularity helped boost his energy.

Having a healthy breakfast along with a consistent morning routine can have a positive ripple effect on the rest of your day. That small success can lead to bigger successes down the road.

I have my own favorite picks for breakfast, but my two top priorities are fiber and protein. They both stabilize blood sugar and keep you full for a long time. For example, you can get protein and fiber in a bowl of oatmeal with chopped walnuts and a side of eggs. There are tons of options to suit your taste. You just have to try them out.

You can also experiment with different ways to boost the protein and fiber in the foods you already eat. Like adding chia seeds to your yogurt and mixing protein powder with hot cereal. Some people enjoy blending a couple tablespoons of chocolate protein powder into their coffee.

If you get stuck in a time crunch, I'd rather you eat on your way to work than skip the meal altogether. This is a great reason to stock up on grab-and-go options. A healthy, frozen burrito (like those from Amy's brand) defrosts quickly in the microwave and you can wrap it in tin foil to take with you. A last resort would be a snack bar you eat on the way. Larabars and Kind bars are two of my favorites because they are made with simple ingredients, typically no more than three or four natural ingredients like nuts and dates.

If you absolutely have no other choice than to go through a drive-through, you can make that work, too. I wouldn't make it a regular habit, but in extreme circumstances you can still make a good choice for yourself. For example, switching to egg sandwiches, like my friend, and avoiding ketchup or other toppings, is still better than skipping breakfast.

The point that I want to drive home for you is that it's incredibly beneficial to have some kind of breakfast each day, even if it's small and quick. The more you develop a pattern of sitting down and slowly eating a hearty breakfast every morning, the better off you will be in the long run. It's not just about the food, either. It's about cultivating habits that are nurturing for optimal health and a balanced body weight. Carving out time for yourself in the morning is essential.

Practical Strategies for BREAKFAST

1. Look at different menus for local drive-throughs and coffee shops that you can use as an emergency back-up for rushed mornings. Research nutrition facts on the menus and find a quick option that prioritizes protein without sugar (think egg sandwich rather than pancakes with syrup). Stay away from juice and high-sugar coffee drinks. Have your sandwich with a simple tea or a small coffee (light on the cream).

2. Plan out your breakfasts the night before or know what you'll be eating for the entire week. Stock up on cartons of egg whites and a hot cereal (sugar-free) that you prefer, such as rolled oats or whole grain toast with eggs.

3. If you hate breakfast or you've just gotten out of the habit, start simple. Try a small, sugar-free (possibly non-dairy) yogurt with fresh strawberry slices or whole grain toast with a light smear of mashed avocado. Find what you like and be consistent.
4. Another quick option is to keep hardboiled eggs, pre-peeled and ready to grab when you are short on time.

STRATEGY 3
The Two-Hour Rule

Once we accept our limits, we go beyond them.
Albert Einstein

This is the only strategy that I categorize as a rule: Stop eating two hours before bedtime. If you are in a calorie deficit and are not eating more calories than your body burns, it technically doesn't matter what time you eat. This is a fact.

So why would I include this two-hour rule and what is the point of it? There are two components to this rule as a practice. One is a physiological component and the other is psychological.

Physiologically, this is related directly to the importance of sleep. Depending on how much food and what type of food you ate last, it can take several hours for that food to digest. Once it leaves your stomach, it needs even more time to further digest and absorb.

Your body works hard to process food, and if you eat right up until bedtime, which many people do, then you're not giving your body the downtime it needs to settle down for rest and recovery. Additionally, if you drink fluids right up until bedtime, you'll likely be waking up to use the bathroom within a few hours, disrupting sleep. When you eat right before you lie down, you also risk indigestion, heartburn, acid reflux, gas, etc. Two hours is an effective time-range to allow your stomach to empty and get far enough into the digestive process, reducing your chances of those issues.

Additionally, two hours is typically not so long that you will get overly hungry prior to bed. If your stomach is grumbling, then that's a sign your dinner was not sufficient. Your last meal should be satisfying and protein-rich so you can avoid snacking into the evening. For example, if you finish eating a sufficient dinner at 7:00 pm and go to bed between 9:00 and 9:30, you will be less likely to have disrupted sleep from either digestive problems or intense hunger.

The other (psychological) component to fasting for two hours before bed is related to building better habits of awareness. This is not deprivation. You are developing awareness related to mindless eating.

When you snack while watching TV or scrolling social media, several handfuls of chips or crackers can add up to a shocking number of empty calories. Setting a hard boundary as a cut-off time for eating makes you aware of maintaining a consistent dinner and sleep schedule. You can have a great day getting in all your balanced meals and snacks but then quickly sabotage yourself by eating hundreds of extra calories while watching a movie. Snacks may seem innocent at the start, but before you know it, you've sabotaged your hard work.

I've had multiple clients respond well to this strategy. One client in particular was a man in his mid-fifties who had great progress with his diet and exercise routine. Then he hit a plateau and began to gain some weight back. I asked him to write down everything he was eating. I recognized a pattern of late-night snacking. He liked eating buttered popcorn with his wife while they watched the ten-o'clock news. I asked him how much he ate, but he couldn't tell me because he was opening a bag and eating until the news was over. Then he would head straight to bed.

It was a tough habit for him to break because it became a pleasant ritual for him and his wife. He took on the challenge, though, and stopped eating two hours before bedtime. His weight dropped back to where he felt his best and he also reported that his nighttime acid reflux went away.

Once you adapt to this strategy and make it a habit, you will appreciate the feeling of going to bed without a big, sluggish belly full of food. You'll wake up well-rested and ready to tackle the day with a positive mindset, having accomplished what you set out to do.

Practical Strategies to APPLY THE TWO-HOUR RULE

1. Determine what time you want to have dinner based on your schedule, as well as what time you want to go to bed. Stick with that plan and be consistent each night.

2. Make sure that dinner is sufficient, including a satisfying protein source (fish, lean turkey, or lean beef). Include fiber from a large portion of vegetables such as asparagus, broccoli, or cauliflower.

3. Include a small portion of healthy fat in your dinner, like a slice of avocado or an ounce of nuts or seeds. Fat digests slowly, which helps you feel satisfied longer.

4. Set an alarm as a reminder to go off at the time your two-hour fasting begins so you create a gentle reminder to stop eating.

5. Keep fluids to a minimum. Take small sips to satisfy thirst but be conscious to avoid big gulps or several glasses of a beverage that could keep you up all night.
6. Set a scheduled time by which you want to be in bed. Start to wind down by keeping the lights dimmed and limiting computer screen time, which can affect your ability to fall asleep. Reading a book in bed is another great way to distract from the urge to snack, and it won't interrupt the sleep cycle.

STRATEGY 4
Fiber

All people are the same; only their habits differ.
Confucius

Adding fiber to your diet is a strategy all on its own. It is one of the absolute best things you can add to your diet on a regular basis. Fiber has so many benefits, one of which being appetite control. It is essential for good health and it's easy to incorporate into your meals. The best part of this strategy is that it focuses on *adding* something to your diet, rather than taking something away. To begin, you should understand the basics of fiber as follows:

There are two types of fiber:

1. **Soluble fiber** is found in things like oats, apples, psyllium, citrus fruits, carrots, and beans. It dissolves in water and helps lower cholesterol and blood sugar levels.

2. **Insoluble fiber**, which is present in beans, vegetables, and nuts, adds bulk to your stool, helping your body to pass a bowel movement.

Fiber is essential for healthy, regular bowel movements, which help prevent issues like hemorrhoids and diverticulitis. By eliminating constipation, your belly feels flatter and intestinal gas is reduced. As an extra bonus, a high fiber diet plays a role in protecting you against colorectal cancer.

Fiber also helps with weight loss. It helps you feel satisfied and full throughout the day because it takes a long time to digest. The more satisfied you feel following a meal, the more likely you are to stick to your eating plan, and that provides the basis for long-term success. Additionally, fiber has positive effects on stabilizing blood sugar.

The current recommendation for daily fiber intake for women is twenty-five grams. For men, it's roughly thirty-eight grams. Because convenience foods are highly processed, most of us aren't even coming close to meeting our needs.

I had a female client once who came to me reluctantly. Her personal trainer convinced her to sign up for nutrition counseling, but she was resistant initially and only came to appease him. I had a tough time trying to figure out how I could help her. Her weight was within a healthy range, but she wanted to improve her overall body composition by modestly reducing body fat. She worked out regularly, but she told me she didn't feel as fit as she'd like. She admitted that she was burnt out on diets and big lifestyle changes that were too disruptive to life with a husband and finicky kids.

I knew she was the perfect example of someone who would benefit more from what I refer to as an *add-in* type of strategy. Add-in strategies refer to something I would add to someone's diet rather than something I would ask them to remove or replace. From a lifestyle perspective, it would prove too challenging for this client to cook differently and swap out her entire pantry of snacks. Because her goals were modest, I felt confident that some reasonable additions could achieve the effect she was looking for.

I asked this client to write a brief overview of her typical day of eating. While she was eating a lot of convenience foods, I saw opportunities where we could boost her fiber. When dietary fiber is adequate and blood sugar levels stabilize, it can help improve mood and energy. It eliminates the need to snack throughout the day and when it's time to sit down for a meal, it's easy to make better choices simply because you don't feel ravenous.

I also gave this client a quick reference guide with all the simple ways to increase fiber in the packaged foods she was already using, such as choosing whole grain or seeded bread in place of white bread. Switching to whole grain pasta is another simple switch. Leaving the skins on potatoes and eggplants as well as fruits like peaches and pears provides an easy boost to fiber content. If you bake homemade applesauce, leave the apple skins on!

I had her add a teaspoon of chia seeds to the yogurt she was already eating most days and she didn't mind having a glass of water mixed with dissolvable fiber (like Metamucil) in the evening after dinner. Whenever she had hot cereal, I had her stir in a tablespoon of psyllium husks, which are tasteless and almost undetectable.

The fiber add-ins were small changes she could live with, and her kids never noticed any difference, which made life easier for her. She was also relieved to discover that she felt better overall and stopped the constant snacking between meals.

A Note on Hormones and Fiber

There is another benefit to increasing your fiber as it relates to hormones. Both men and women produce estrogen, just at different levels. When estrogen levels are too high, however, it not only affects hormone balance, but it can also lead to weight gain, irregular periods, mood swings, and irritability. Estrogen is also produced in fat cells. So, the more body fat we carry, the more likely we are to have excess estrogen. Nevertheless, the body can eliminate excess estrogen through regular bowel movements.

A diet high in fiber helps us produce regular bowel movements, thus aiding the elimination of the estrogen surplus by way of excretion. Excess estrogen exits through the bowels, and if you don't produce stool every day, then that excess hormone remains in the colon and can get reabsorbed into our body, which *could* contribute to an imbalance.

There is one caveat to adding fiber to your diet, at least in the early stages. Be aware that as you increase your daily fiber intake, you may initially experience some temporary gas and bloating. If that is the case, simply back off a little and add the fiber more gradually.

How well you tolerate the increase in fiber all depends on your current diet, and to some degree, the health status of your digestion. Any initial gas or bloating will resolve with time and patience. I also cannot overstate the importance of adequate water intake. If you increase your fiber and you're chronically dehydrated, you can wind up with constipation. Remember that fiber adds bulk to your stool, but without enough water, it will not eliminate smoothly.

Practical Strategies for FIBER

1. Add more fresh fruits and vegetables to your diet, such as fresh strawberries or blackberries in your morning cereal. Have roasted or steamed veggies with every lunch and dinner, or a fresh salad as your appetizer.
2. Include a spoonful of psyllium husk flakes or chia seeds in your hot cereal or yogurt.
3. Make a morning or afternoon smoothie and add a cup of fresh spinach or kale.
4. Establish an evening protocol following dinner, using dissolvable fiber mixed in water (such as Metamucil or Renew Life Clear Fiber). Follow the recommended dosage on the label.

STRATEGY 5
The Vegetable Edge

To eat is a necessity, but to eat intelligently is an art.
F. De La Rochefoucauld

If you ask most people to list their favorite foods, you're not likely to see vegetables near the top of the list. Most of us hated vegetables as kids and, unfortunately, carried that distaste into adulthood.

Veggies can seem boring when compared with something like lasagna or cheeseburgers, but the reality is that vegetables, when prepared correctly, are food superstars *and* they contain a secret special power. Not only are veggies loaded with vitamins, minerals, and antioxidants, they are also amazingly fiber-rich while being (mostly) low in calories. This quality is their superpower because they can add tons of volume to a meal with little caloric impact *and* major nutrient density!

Salads have the potential to be a rich source of vegetables. Sadly, the perception of "diet foods" and salads go hand in hand. Ironically, though, most of the salads I see on restaurant menus are loaded with fat and calories making them the worst choice if you're trying to eat healthy. Restaurant salads are typically loaded with things like croutons, cheese, tortilla strips, and rich salad dressings, which are best to avoid altogether.

I personally love salads to boost my daily vegetable intake, but I make them at home with the right ingredients to keep them as healthy as possible. When it comes to helping others with their diet, though, I usually don't push salads because of the diet stigma associated with them.

With most of the people I've counseled over the years, I look for other creative ways to get them to include more vegetables in their diet. Many clients have cringed when I've asked them to have vegetables at every lunch and dinner. The key to changing their minds is helping them understand that veggies are incredibly filling. Satiety is always one of the *primary* determinants of success.

I have a female friend who is a busy physician. She had little spare time to incorporate an exercise regimen and she didn't have the energy to make a lot of dietary changes. What she did do, however, was add vegetables in large quantities to two of her main meals every day. She allowed herself to eat as many vegetables as she wanted. That's all she did, and she lost over thirty pounds! That's an impressive testimonial for vegetables.

Palatability is often the main obstacle. You must find preparation methods that work for you. It's also necessary to find substitute toppings and dressings that aren't overly fattening. Avoid creamy dressings like ranch and blue cheese. Don't cook vegetables with heavy amounts of butter or oil. Prepare veggies steamed, grilled, or roasted and stay away from anything fried or breaded.

For home-baked meals specifically, the most reliable strategy for increasing your veggie intake is to prepare everything in advance or "meal prep." Meal prepping is basically when you finish your shopping, come home, and wash and cut your vegetables or salad mixes. Then you cook up a huge batch that will last the entire week. When everything is pre-prepared, you only need to reheat. An air fryer is a great way to reheat and restore a crispy texture to vegetables.

I cover meal prep thoroughly in a later chapter. In the meantime, look for creative ways to add some greens to your meals. It can be as simple as sautéing some spinach in the same pan you cook your protein. Or mix minced onions and peppers into lean ground beef patties.

If you are motivated to include salads, that's great. The benefits of the raw, healthy greens are amazing, but be aware of the very high calories in most dressings. Look for light versions and pay attention to the serving size (which is typically 2 tablespoons).

Fibrous vegetables can be eaten in almost unlimited quantities because they are very low in calories and high in fiber. They include veggies like spinach, asparagus, broccoli, brussels sprouts, cauliflower, cucumber, celery, onions, peppers, and zucchini.

Starchy vegetables are higher in calories and carbohydrates and can still be included in your meal plan but in measured amounts. Some popular starchy vegetables include corn, potatoes, butternut squash, sweet potatoes, yams, and peas. Keep these to a minimum while loading up on the fibrous vegetables to maximize the volume of food you eat at each meal.

Green Smoothies

Green smoothies are a great way to pack a bunch of veggies into a condensed, portable shake, but I would caution against commercially bought versions from the grocery store or a smoothie shop. Those are made to maximize flavor and often include high amounts of nut butters, fruits, juice, and syrups, making them very high in calories. Additionally, the store-bought versions tend to be low in fiber and you won't stay full for very long. In a similar way, fresh-pressed juices are problematic because all the fiber has been removed in the juicing process.

The best green smoothies are the ones that use water or a low-calorie base such as unsweetened almond milk. They are packed with spinach, kale, or other leafy greens like Swiss chard. Other healthy additives include hemp hearts, flax seeds, avocado, and protein powder. Low-calorie sweeteners like stevia or monk fruit can add sweetness.

If you plan to drink some smoothies each week, purchase a high-powered blender to pulverize the fibrous greens into a smooth, creamy texture. I also recommend purchasing your ingredients in advance and having them ready to use. Large bags of frozen berries and bananas help with preparation and the frozen fruit enhances the texture of the shake. There are a lot of great recipes online for tasty smoothies, but I recommend sticking with a foundation of ingredients that include *a protein source, a healthy fat*, and some type of *berry* and *leafy greens*. The following is a basic recipe I like to use, and I rotate the source of greens and berries each week (one week I might use spinach and strawberries, then the next week use kale and blackberries, etc.):

Base Green Smoothie Recipe

(This recipe easily fits into a large 64-ounce Vitamix blender)

- 2 cups fresh, cold water or 1 cup unsweetened almond milk (add additional water as needed for texture)
- ½ banana (frozen)
- 1 heaping cup raw, organic spinach (or kale)
- 1/3 cup blackberries (frozen)
- 1 heaping scoop of your favorite protein powder (I prefer Casein protein powder)
- A dash of powdered stevia
- ¼ avocado (frozen) or 1 tablespoon raw almond butter

Optional additions to the base recipe:

- 1 tablespoon ground flaxseeds / 1 tablespoon hemp hearts / 1 tablespoon chia seeds

Practical Strategies for INCREASING VEGETABLES AND NUTRIENT DENSITY

1. Find creative recipes that use vegetables in a way that "hides" them with flavor. For example, mixing equal parts spaghetti squash with regular pasta can be integrated into a pasta dish while maintaining the same flavor and texture of spaghetti and meatballs. You can use zucchini noodles in a similar way.
2. Experiment with canned pureed pumpkin, mashed bananas, or sugar-free applesauce in quick breads and muffins as a healthy substitute for the fat that the recipe calls for. These are obviously fruits, but this approach utilizes the same concept for increasing nutrient density in your homemade dishes.
3. Blend a handful of spinach into almost any smoothie to camouflage the taste.
4. Smear mashed avocado in place of any type of spread on a sandwich or wrap.
5. Make any kind of ground meat entrée (like meatloaf) with finely chopped veggies mixed in.
6. Cook a batch of sugar-free applesauce using monk fruit/ lakanto as a sweet side dish.

7. Pre-purchase smoothie ingredients and freeze (or purchase them frozen). Frozen avocado chunks will ensure that avocados never turn bad and go to waste.
8. Buy a shaker bottle for smoothies to keep the ingredients from settling at the bottom of the container.
9. Stock up on large bags of berries in the freezer section at your local big box store.
10. Peel and freeze browning bananas to store in the freezer for smoothies.

STRATEGY 6
Protein Strategies

Day by day, what you choose, what you think,
and what you do is who you become.
Heraclitus

Protein must be one of your priorities when it comes to weight loss or body composition changes. It is likely you are not getting enough protein in your diet to support your goals. What makes protein so special? One reason is that, like fiber, protein is very filling and satiating. It will make you less susceptible to unplanned snacking and bingeing.

Protein is one of three "macro" nutrients your body needs to complete its functions and provide the structural components in our tissues and organs. It also plays a role in supporting the growth and maintenance of muscle tissue. Muscle has a direct relationship to our metabolism. The more muscle you have, the more calories you burn. This is one reason why weight-bearing exercise is so effective in developing overall health and fitness.

I have had more than a few female clients who have struggled with this concept. I recall one female client who was adamant that she did not want to "bulk up." She equated the idea of eating more protein with becoming muscled up. This is simply not possible, but I had a hard time convincing her. People sometimes associate high-protein diets and protein powders with bodybuilders. So, it wasn't uncommon that I would encounter this concern with some clients. I can assure you, though, that you would need to lift *very* heavy weights for several years to add significant muscle to your body. It would take a concerted effort.

I had to ask this particular client for her blind faith. I knew that if she just followed the instructions I gave her, she would understand. We agreed to a short trial period of two weeks so she would have a chance to experience the benefits. She made the commitment, and within days, she started to reap the rewards of feeling increased stamina and a reduced urge to snack. She felt energized for her daily walks and told me after the fact that, to her relief, she felt stronger without noticing any of the bulkiness she worried about. I was happy she was willing to give it a try.

If you're not used to eating a high-protein diet, you might struggle to find ways of adding it to your meals. There are plenty of excellent high-protein foods, and the more variety you include, the less likely you are to be bored.

Some great protein sources include:

- Wild caught fish
- Seafood (scallops, shrimp, lobster)
- Lean cuts of beef (ground beef, eye of round, sirloin tip, top round)
- Elk and bison
- Chicken and turkey (skinless, white meat poultry and 98–99% lean-ground versions)
- Whole eggs and egg whites (which you can buy in cartons)
- Dairy products (if you tolerate them) like cottage cheese and low-fat yogurt
- Lean pork (tenderloin)

In addition to meat, poultry, and fish, you can try protein powders as a more convenient source of protein. They are excellent for travel and when you need a quick meal or snack. You can purchase a shaker bottle, which allows you to dump a scoop or two of protein powder in it to stash in your car or work bag. When you are ready for it, just add water and shake it up. In a pinch, it's very efficient.

How to choose a protein powder

The best protein powder is the one that tastes the best to you. If you hate the taste, you'll never use it, and it will sit on a shelf doing you no good. Luckily, protein powders have improved dramatically over the years and there are many options to choose from. Whenever possible, get sample sizes to try before buying a large container and choose the flavors that are most appealing to you. It really doesn't matter too much whether you use egg white protein, casein, or whey. It's more important that you like the flavor and texture and that it digests easily.

Some powders have sweeteners like sucralose, which can cause gas and bloating for some people. If that is the case, then look for a natural sweetener like stevia or monk fruit. It might not be as sweet, but it should digest better for you. If you are lactose intolerant, you may need to avoid whey and casein powders since they are by-products of dairy. Plant-based protein powders can be a good option, as well.

Other things to consider when looking at protein powders are, of course, the number of calories, fat, and protein in a serving size, which is typically one scoop. Here are some general guidelines to look for in one serving size:

- Calories no greater than 120–150 calories per serving/scoop
- Protein should ideally be a minimum of twenty grams per serving (20-25 grams is a good range)
- Less than five grams of sugar (less is better)

- Fiber content is a bonus, and if you can find a protein with three grams or more, that's great

Some protein powders will even add probiotics, greens, and digestive enzymes. The extras aren't necessary, but they may provide some benefit.

Something worth mentioning is that it's not ideal to have more than one shake a day (except in circumstances where you are unable to have all your regular meals). It is always best to have real, whole foods. You should eat complete meals as much as possible. Protein shakes are mostly for convenience and times when you just can't fit in a proper meal.

How much protein should I be eating?

I will cover this question in greater detail in the chapter on macros and macro counting. But a good place to start, generally speaking, is between twenty to thirty grams of protein in each meal.

Practical Strategies for PROTEIN

1. Keep a stockpile of beef jerky or meat sticks on hand for quick protein snacks on the go.
2. Look for hardboiled eggs in convenience stores in a pinch or keep some stored at home.
3. Keep cartons of egg whites in the refrigerator when you need to boost the protein in your breakfast (for example, cooking up two whole eggs and adding in extra egg whites will keep the calories in check while boosting the protein and volume).

4. Have nuts available in your pantry. They are very calorie-dense and not the best source of protein but are still nutritious and filling. They can easily be found in convenience stores if you find yourself hungry on the road.
5. Store protein powder in a zip-lock bag in your car. Just grab a bottle of water and mix with the powder in an emergency.
6. Keep a small cooler in your car or travel bag with beef jerky and snacks.
7. Shop for protein bars that are low in sugar and high in fiber.
8. Determine your protein goals when you get to the chapter on macros, then plan your meals accordingly.

STRATEGY 7
Eat More to Eat Less

If one oversteps the bounds of moderation,
the greatest pleasures cease to please.
Epictetus

One of the keys to making healthier choices is to make absolute sure you never get so hungry that you overeat all the wrong foods. Starving your way through the day leaves you miserable, cranky, and weak-willed. It leads to fattening drive-through food on the way home from work and impulse binges. Being ravenous is never a good thing and it is completely unsustainable.

Over the years, I've heard clients and friends talk about "saving up" for big events. For example, I had a client who liked to eat very lightly before holiday parties and weddings. She thought she was saving calories so she could eat what she wanted at her event. However, it always backfired (and usually does). She'd arrive hungry and fill up on alcohol and appetizers because she couldn't wait for the main meal. The night typically ended as a binging disaster. She'd come into my office afterwards feeling miserable, like she had ruined her progress. The guilt of these common scenarios is almost worse than the actual mishap, leading to a defeatist mindset and discouragement. Unfortunately, it's not uncommon.

It honestly took me years to really get this concept, too. I didn't want to trust the process and follow it through. I resisted large, filling meals at breakfast, lunch, and dinner. I wanted to skimp at my main meals so that I would have some surplus at the end of the day to indulge the cravings I always had after dinner. I thought if I saved up for the end of the day, then I could still have a big dessert. However, I had it completely backwards and it wasn't the healthiest approach. It affected my energy levels and my mood. Once I surrendered to eating more and making sure I had satisfying meals, I suddenly realized my intense sugar cravings subsided.

When I balanced my meals with plenty of protein, fiber, and veggies, I immediately noticed that because I was satiated, my cravings faded significantly. I do still have a sweet treat after dinner, but the endless cravings finally let up. The more consistent I was with having a healthy portion of nutrient-dense food, the less I felt gripped by cravings throughout the day. I never save up for events like Thanksgiving, either. It's fine if you want to eat a little lighter if you know an extra-large meal is around the corner, but never starve yourself.

Planning your meals and some scheduled snacks takes some thought and preparation. You don't want to leave things to chance. Aim to eat a meal or snack every three to four hours, and once you establish this practice, it becomes routine, and you'll never be hangry again!

I recommend keeping items at your desk at work as well as in your purse, and even consider keeping a small cooler in your car for snacks. I've also listed several ideas on emergency food in the appendixes. Back-up snacks have saved me when I have been stuck in traffic or when appointments run long. Healthy, available snacks keep you sane on busy days, and your energy and mood stay even and steady.

The following is an example of well-timed snacks and meals:

6:30 am: Breakfast

9:30 am: Mid-morning snack (if needed)

12:00 pm: Lunch

3:00 pm: Afternoon snack

6:30 pm: Dinner

A good snack choice is approximately 250 calories or less and rich in protein. Your main meals will be a bit larger and should include whole, unprocessed foods. A common complaint about frequent eating is that there are days when things get busy and either the snacks are forgotten or there is no time to stop and eat.

Overall, consistency is most important. Don't worry about misses here and there; eating your main meals takes priority. The snacks are there in case you do get hungry in between or if one of your main meals is delayed or skipped unintentionally. For instance, if a meeting runs late or you get stuck in a traffic jam, having a snack available will prevent intense cravings and bingeing later in the day.

Practical Strategies for EATING MORE TO EAT LESS

1. Review the "Macros, Prepping, and Tracking" chapter to determine how much protein you should eat per day on average. Divide that total by the number of meals you plan to eat and aim to reach that goal consistently.
2. Include a serving of vegetables at every lunch and dinner. If you choose fibrous veggies like asparagus, broccoli, or cauliflower, eat as much as you like.

3. Add fiber to hot cereal in the morning by stirring in a heaping tablespoon of psyllium husk flakes and/or a teaspoon of chia seeds. They both add bulk to your cereal and increase satiety.
4. Use antioxidant-packed berries like strawberries, raspberries, blackberries, and blueberries to add to hot cereal or yogurt. They boost nutrition and add volume to your snack or meal.
5. Increase the volume of protein and veggies in your meals when you feel exceptionally hungry. You can eat more of these with minimal impact on calories.
6. Manage cravings by including a small amount of your guilty pleasures into your planned meal. For example, if you're at a dinner party buffet and you've made your plate of healthy choices, but you're craving the lasagna, then add a small portion of it to your plate. You will satisfy your cravings, but you'll be full, preventing you from going back for seconds.
7. Eating more to eat less is about having a small snack just prior to special events like holiday parties or weddings where you don't know what options you'll be given. While you're on your way to the event, have something like a meat stick or an ounce of nuts. Then you won't be tempted to gorge on hors d'oeuvres, bread baskets, and alcohol. It will feel counterintuitive, but you'll consume fewer calories in the long run.

The Following is an example day of meals and snacks that utilizes several volume-enhancing strategies. Please keep in mind that you will need to choose your own meals and snacks based on your individual macros as well as your preferred tastes and preferences.

Breakfast:

1/3 cup oatmeal

1 cup egg whites plus 1 whole egg (cooked with non-stick pan spray)

1 tablespoon psyllium husk flakes

1/3 cup raspberries

Mid-Morning Snack:

1 ounce mixed nuts (pistachios and raw cashews)

Lunch:

3 ounces grilled skinless chicken breast

2 slices whole grain bread

Lettuce, tomato, and mustard

1 cup steamed broccoli

Afternoon Snack:

2 meat sticks *or* 1 container low-fat Greek yogurt *or* 1–2 hard-boiled eggs

Dinner:

3 ounces grilled salmon

1–2 cups grilled asparagus

½ baked potato

2 pieces dark chocolate

STRATEGY 8
Gut Health: Eliminating What Doesn't Work

Let food be thy medicine…
Hippocrates

If you've ever suffered with digestive issues, then you are well aware of how important gut health is. Food sensitivities and gut problems seem to be rampant. The average American might be surprised to learn that sixty-five percent of the population is lactose intolerant. Research suggests that it is a genetic anomaly to tolerate milk as an adult, which seems shocking considering the number of dairy products on shelves. Celiac disease and gluten intolerance are a growing issue, as well.

Many people discover immediate relief once they eliminate dairy and/or gluten for a few weeks. They don't realize that it's the source of their digestive problems until after they've removed it from their diet. Regardless of the culprit, if you have digestive upset on a regular basis, you need to identify the cause and eliminate the problem. There's no guarantee that eliminating a particular food group will help you lose weight, but I have seen it happen.

I had a friend who had a moderate weight problem that he was working on through diet and exercise. His progress was sluggish, at best, but he only began to see significant results when he cut gluten out of his diet completely. I am not suggesting that gluten avoidance is a strategy to lose weight. Rather, people who experience major digestive issues with certain food groups seem to have an easier time with weight loss once they have identified the irritant and eliminated it. After only a few weeks of eating a gluten-free diet, he noticed improved sleep, more energy, and his weight loss became more consistent and substantial.

The moral of the story is that when food isn't digesting well, it's a sign that your body is struggling to function properly. Your digestive tract can become inflamed as it struggles to eliminate food that does not agree with you, and if you're not processing food efficiently, chances are your body can't function optimally.

My personal experience with food intolerance began in my twenties. It felt as though all the foods I ate as a teenager were suddenly giving me issues. I ate plenty of bread and cheese while growing up, but I could no longer eat things like ice cream without a major backlash. And it only continued to worsen with age. When a family member was diagnosed with Celiac disease, I decided to go gluten-free myself. It took several weeks to notice a difference, but I came to recognize a dramatic improvement in my gut health while avoiding not only gluten, but dairy, as well. I've never noticed any change in my weight directly related to abstaining from irritating foods, but the absence of digestive problems has been so positive that I'll never go back. My whole body feels better when my gut health is in check.

Gluten and dairy are two well-known culprits when it comes to digestive issues, but there are other foods that commonly give people trouble, as well. FODMAP is an acronym that simply refers to a group of carbohydrates that are resistant to digestion and end up causing gas and bloating. Dairy (which has lactose) is part of the FODMAPS group. Other foods in this group include onions, garlic, legumes and sugar alcohols like xylitol, mannitol, and sorbitol (which are found in many "sugar-free" products).

While it is important to look out for foods that cause you trouble, it's also helpful to support your gut health with probiotics or probiotic-rich foods. Fermented foods are naturally rich in probiotics, and it is valuable to add them to your daily diet. I have at least one meal with them every day.

Foods such as kimchi, miso, and sauerkraut are fermented and easy to find in most stores. If you're someone who tolerates dairy, kefir and yogurt naturally contain probiotics. Most non-dairy yogurts have probiotics, as well. Additionally, adequate fiber and hydration contribute significantly to a healthy gut.

If you've tried everything else and still have problems, consider food-combining principles. Proponents of food combining suggest that based on a food's composition and digestibility, that food may or may not digest thoroughly if eaten with non-compatible foods. For example, fruit tends to digest more quickly than meat, so if you eat a bowl of cantaloupe (which digests more quickly) immediately after a meat-rich meal (which digests more slowly) you may experience problems because the fruit is sitting in your gut for a long time waiting for the meat to be digested. There is really no research on food combining, so this approach is based solely on anecdotal evidence, but some people who use the combining principles (including myself) report positive results, and it may be worth trying.

Food-Combining Principles:

1. Eat fruit alone on an empty stomach.
2. Eat proteins with non-starchy, fibrous vegetables (leafy greens, broccoli, cabbage, cauliflower, lettuce, zucchini, cucumber). No proteins with starches.
3. Eat starchy vegetables and grains with non-starchy vegetables (starchy vegetables include squash, peas, corn, lima beans, potatoes).

4. Fats and oils can be eaten with grains, vegetables, and protein.

Another consideration is how we affect the process of digestion through our actions and physical, emotional, and mental state while eating. We digest foods two ways:

1. Mechanical (chewing)
2. Chemical (digestive enzymes and hydrochloric acid)

Consciously make an effort to chew your food thoroughly before swallowing for better digestion. Don't eat while distracted with social media, work, or TV. Relax and savor your food and remove any distractions that make you feel anxious or stressed while eating.

Practical Strategies for GUT HEALTH

1. Try aged cheese (which has little to no lactose after the ageing process) if you need to eliminate dairy but still crave cheese. Try a vegan or plant-based cheese alternative.
2. Use goat's milk or sheep's milk yogurts as dairy alternatives.
3. Add in a daily probiotic.
4. Add sauerkraut, kimchi and kombucha to meals to boost probiotics.
5. Drink lots of water (at least three liters per day) to help with overall digestive health and efficiency.
6. Consider taking digestive enzymes with your meals.
7. Create a peaceful space to eat calmly and slowly, and don't forget to chew your food thoroughly.

STRATEGY 9
Eliminate Alcohol

If you want more, you have to require more from yourself.
Phil McGraw

Alcohol plays a big role in our social lives. We associate it with celebration, time spent with friends, and a simple way to relax at the end of a hard day. Unfortunately, even in moderate amounts, alcohol has negative effects on your best effort to reach your goals. It is a major obstacle to weight loss, which is why this strategy is so important to your success.

For context, here is a brief overview of how alcohol compares to the other primary nutrients:

- Protein has four calories per gram.
- Carbohydrates have four calories per gram.
- Fat has nine calories per gram.
- Alcohol has seven calories per gram.

Alcohol contains almost as many calories as fat, but it doesn't fill you up. It also falls into the "liquid calories" category, except it's worse than other types of liquid calories. Unlike something like juice, alcohol has *zero* nutritional value...not even a single vitamin! However, the worst effect of alcohol is that it lowers your inhibitions and your resolve to make good choices. That means you are much more likely to go way off track and eat things that don't serve you or your goals. Drinking alcohol also affects you the next day; it's dehydrating and can give you a hangover, or severe headache, which is likely to make you cancel the workout you had planned. Even one glass of wine can leave you feeling like you'd rather sleep in than get up and go to the gym.

An average serving size of red wine, for example, has 123 calories, but the "average" glass is considered five ounces or 148 grams. Five ounces is just a little more than a quarter of a cup, which is tiny! It is more likely you get six ounces or more per glass, which equates to roughly 142 calories. In other words, having two glasses of wine adds up to approximately 284 calories! If you average two glasses of wine three times per week, that's about 852 extra calories per week.

Since alcohol is dehydrating and dehydration can mimic hunger, you'll likely eat more than you might otherwise. Alcohol also disturbs sleep patterns, which means you won't get a good night of sleep, and when you don't get your eight hours, you release more of the *appetite-stimulating* hormone, ghrelin. Additionally, drinking alcohol can affect metabolic rate and disrupt the production of testosterone, which is present in men and women, affecting your ability to burn calories efficiently.

This is a tough strategy to embrace. Clients I've had put up hard resistance when I've approached this topic. A male client I worked with years ago started our sessions with enthusiasm and eagerness to learn about nutrition until the topic of eliminating alcohol came up. His passion for learning turned into hostility. I was certain he was going to quit, and I'd never see him again. This was a typical response, though. For most of the clients I've worked with, I've discovered that their opposition is typically grounded in fear. Lots of people have social anxiety that is alleviated by alcohol, or they have fears rooted in social pressure they anticipate from friends and family.

Your fear or hesitancy might feel valid, but only you can find your "why." The why is your reason for wanting to change your eating habits in the first place. That's the determining factor when things get difficult.

My client didn't quit my services, after all. We talked about his goals and why he was spending money to come see me each week for nutrition counseling. It turned out that his deep desire to live a healthier life carried enough weight to give him the strength of commitment to those goals. He realized his attachment to alcohol was not as rewarding as the progress he made once he gave it up completely. It was a time of transformation for him, as it has been for many of my clients. It's the moment you realize that some of the things you are holding onto are the same things holding you back. Never let a temporary pleasure like alcohol take precedence over a lifetime of the freedom you feel when you master your goals.

Alcohol is tempting, but it will never be worth ruining your efforts and creating constant setbacks for yourself. Once you get alcohol out of your life, a whole new world opens up to you. You discover new places to go and different things to do. Your social circle expands to include new people and you realize there was nothing to fear in the first place.

If you make the decision to put your health first, set a short-term goal to eliminate alcohol for sixty days. See how you feel and notice what happens with your weight. Sixty days is an easy time frame to put something to the test. In the meantime, plan different things to do on the weekends that don't involve alcohol. Make a list of different things to try instead of going out for drinks. This is a transformative strategy on so many levels if you're willing to give yourself the time and attention to put it into practice.

Practical Strategies to ELIMINATE ALCOHOL

1. Make a list of the pros and cons of drinking alcohol and see how the two columns stack up against each other. A pro might be that you have an easier time socializing, but one of the cons might be that you miss your workout the next day.
2. Do an online search for fun things to do in your area. You might discover lots of opportunities to check out new places and activities where you can meet friends that don't involve alcohol.
3. Join an online group of like-minded people who organize regular gatherings for activities like hikes with their dogs or snowshoeing.
4. Talk to your friends and family and let them know that you are abstaining from alcohol. You'll quickly discover who is supportive and who is not, so you can choose to spend time with the ones who encourage you.

STRATEGY 10
Estrogens and Obesogens

Prevention is better than cure.
Desiderius Erasmus

This strategy addresses *potentially* harmful additives in our foods and environment and how to best avoid them. This is an area of emerging scientific data and is speculative, but it's worth incorporating into your lifestyle. Most studies on chemical additives, like the one supported by the National Institutes of Health in 2012, have only been based on animal research. But over the years, researchers have noted that lab animals gain weight when exposed to chemical additives that are currently found in many household products and foods.

Scientists who focus their studies on factors affecting obesity have identified what are now referred to as *obesogens*. Obesogens are chemically derived "endocrine disruptors." The endocrine system encompasses many glands and organs in the body and includes the hormones they secrete. Hormones are chemical messengers that control and regulate cell and organ activity. The impact of hormone imbalance can have widespread and damaging consequences on your body. I touched briefly on the impacts of excess estrogen in the chapter on fiber, but this chapter helps you systematically identify and remove sources of potential hormone-disrupting ingredients that hide in your environment and *possibly* interfere with your weight-loss efforts.

Hormones play a role in everything from growth and sexual development to immune response, metabolism, sleep cycles, and insulin release, to name a few endocrine functions. New evidence suggests environmental factors may be contributing to some of the weight problems many adults and children struggle with. Obesogens include any natural or man-made chemical that mimics the hormones in our body. This mimicking of hormones prevents our naturally occurring hormones from acting correctly.

Potential Sources of Obesogens

- BPA – a synthetic estrogen found in the plastic bottles we drink our water from; the lining of certain canned foods; medical devices; cash register receipts.
- PFOA (perfluorooctanoic acid) – a surfactant used for friction reduction and found in non-stick cook ware, carpets, furniture, waterproof clothing, microwave popcorn bags, and pizza boxes.
- Pesticides – on food products as well as in some tap water, as pesticides leach into the soil and enter our water sources.
- Phthalates – used in shower curtains, air fresheners, and plastic wrap, as well as some body care items like lotions, creams, and nail polish.
- Parabens – found in many personal care items such as lotions, shampoos, creams, and make-up.

Foods that May Increase Estrogen

- *Large* amounts of caffeine (3 or more cups of coffee per day).
- Foods high in fat and sugar.

- Alcohol – even moderate alcohol consumption is associated with increased estrogen levels and decreased testosterone levels.
- A Diet Low in Fiber – while a high-fiber diet helps eliminate excess estrogen, conversely a low-fiber diet allows it to proliferate.
- Dairy Products – because dairy cows lactate, their hormones are high during the milking process which means their estrogen levels are high and transferred into the milk products we consume.
- Soy – the verdict is still out. There are presently studies and commentaries that support the idea that soy may be problematic when it comes to estrogen. So, at this point moderation is the best guideline when considering soy product consumption. Choose organic to be extra safe and always refer to the American Cancer Society research for the latest findings.

Ultimately, there is a lot to consider when it comes to cleaning up your home environment and food choices in relation to potentially unhealthy chemicals. You can do research when buying new products to make healthier choices. You can also make some gradual, common-sense modifications to your diet such as eating organic when possible. And consider purchases you make in body care and cleaning products. This may help make an improvement in how many obesogens and chemicals you're exposed to on a daily basis. A diet high in fiber is an excellent place to start as well as eliminating dairy and alcohol, as mentioned above. Also, take care to replace your water bottles with the BPA-free kinds (most bottles are now labeled if they are BPA-free) or purchase a stainless-steel bottle.

There are excellent resources online to help you make safer choices in lotions, make-up, and household cleaners with ingredient lists. Look for labels on the packaging which clearly state that the product is free of parabens, phthalates, sodium laurel sulfate, etc. to eliminate the additives, which are potentially unhealthy and unnecessary. We can't possibly eliminate all the toxins from our lives. But I believe it is a worthwhile precaution to limit your exposure.

I don't have examples of clients who could definitively conclude that they reached weight loss goals by simply eliminating certain household products. It is impossible to measure the effects of making those changes, unless someone in your family has, for example, allergies that were relieved by eliminating certain additives. I *have* had clients, though, who felt better after they began to scrutinize the products they used. For example, one client realized that once she eliminated fragrances in her household products, her regular headaches began to subside. She just hadn't realized she was sensitive to artificial scents.

Another client had a son with asthma. She noticed he was using his inhaler less frequently several months after she changed most of the home products she was buying. This is an area of growing research and concern, and it's worth considering the chemical load you place on your body. Many small details within your lifestyle can add up to big impacts over the course of many years. When you care about your health, seek to play the long game, and consider the cumulative effects of everything in your lifestyle and environment.

Practical Strategies to ADDRESS ESTROGENS AND OBESOGENS

1. Avoid cooking food in plastic containers. The chemicals in the plastic, when heated, can leach into your food. Instead, transfer the food into a glass or stainless-steel pan before re-heating.
2. Limit buying food and drink products that use plastic packaging (like bottled water).
3. Buy body care products that are labeled as phthalate- and paraben-free.
4. Avoiding non-stick cookware (which contains chemicals that can leach into food) and choose cast iron, stainless-steel, and glass instead.
5. Choose organic foods whenever possible.
6. Swap out household detergents and cleaners to environmentally friendly versions that avoid using harsh chemicals and perfumes.
7. Wash and rinse produce. Make your own vegetable wash by mixing one cup vinegar with four cups of water and storing in a spray bottle.

STRATEGY 11
The Extras

Good habits are the key to all success.
Bad habits are the unlocked door to failure.
Og Mandino

Condiments, dips, sauces, marinades, and added sugars…these are all the extras that go unaccounted for. These items are also the reason that navigating restaurant food is so tricky; it's hard to know exactly how many extra calories you get with sauces and condiments, and it's tough to make an accurate guess. Take ketchup, for example. There are roughly twenty calories in a tablespoon of standard ketchup, and if you dip French fries in it, a tablespoon might only cover two or three fries at most. You could easily consume several hundred calories in ketchup alone with a small serving of fries.

If extras like sauces and dressings aren't accounted for, you can easily add way more fat, sugar, and calories than you are aware of. This is not to say that everything you eat must be dry and flavorless, but it is important to make better choices and find alternatives. Ketchup has always been one of my favorite condiments and I like to put in on everything. It's loaded with sugar, though, so I looked around and found a few sugar-free brands I really like. It saves a ton of excess calories and I still get to enjoy my ketchup!

I had a female client once who, after having a baby the year before, struggled to get back in shape. She was super motivated to reach her goals and she jumped into our sessions with both feet. Everything seemed to be on point. She was exercising regularly and incorporating all the adjustments I made to her eating habits. She had great success and lost weight at a steady pace. Her commitment was inspiring. However, we got to a point about five months in when she began to plateau. Her weight didn't budge for several weeks in a row, and she grew frustrated. I asked her to keep a journal of everything she ate for one week so I could identify the culprit. When we sat down together and dug into the details, I realized what was getting in the way of her continued progress.

All the extras that added up each day halted her momentum. We talked about the regular bites of food she took off her toddler's plate, the condiments that had hidden sugars, and the mindless habit of munching on the food she was preparing for meals. She hadn't been aware of the extras that went unaccounted for. It was a lightbulb moment for her. It never occurred to her that all those little details could have such an impact.

I gave her ideas for healthier alternatives to her condiments and marinades, and I made sure her main meals were filling enough that she didn't need to grab bites here and there. The realization was enough for her to turn things around and get her progress moving forward again. She eventually exceeded her goals and went on to become a fitness instructor. No doubt, she and her family were much healthier for her tremendous efforts.

When it comes to accounting for the extras, it can be a bit of a turn-off to see the importance of every detail, but the fact is that modern food has strayed far from its origins. Almost everything that is on a shelf or in a package has been altered in some way. Processed food has tons of sugar, flavorings, and colors added. We get so many extra calories and junk added to our food that if you don't look at everything comprehensively, you will hit the same roadblocks my client had and never truly understand why your efforts seem fruitless.

The extras are an obstacle almost every one of my clients encountered at some point during their journey. The details matter. The good news is that food manufacturing has expanded dramatically over the last decade. There are endless manufacturers who pride themselves on sourcing the best ingredients, making it much easier to find healthier alternatives. Getting clear on the details equals *freedom*!

The following is a list of condiments that are great "as is." They are naturally low in calories and fat:

- Mustard (almost all types)
- Salt, pepper, and herbs
- Salsa
- Vinegars (Balsamic, apple cider vinegar, etc.)
- Hot sauces
- Teriyaki and soy sauces (look for low-sodium versions)
- Sugar-free Barbecue sauce
- Braggs liquid Aminos (tastes very similar to soy sauce)
- Sugar-free ketchup
- Lite versions of salad dressings (can also be used as marinades)
- Lemon juice (as a marinade for chicken)
- Horseradish
- Tomato sauces (sugar-free options are easy to find)
- Nutritional yeast (as a topping that has a "cheesy" flavor)

You can also get creative when cooking with condiments by blending different flavors. For example, if you love tuna fish for sandwiches, there are alternatives to standard mayonnaise. Look for a light mayo *or* you can mix the light mayonnaise with equal parts of hummus. Hummus has more nutritional value and it's lower in calories than standard mayo. You can also try using hummus by itself and see if you like the flavor. Some online recipe browsing can help you discover new ways of enjoying the foods you love without the excess calories.

Sugar

It's important to consider the added sugar in the foods you eat. Sugar is not good or bad, per say. The problem with sugar is that it has no nutritional value and it's added to almost all processed foods. This adds a tremendous number of additional calories.

Sugar comes in many forms. It might be listed in the ingredients as high-fructose corn syrup, maltose, fructose, sucrose, dextrose, or malt syrup. You also might see the sugar listed as maple syrup, molasses, honey, fruit juice concentrate, brown sugar, or cane crystals. They're all processed in the body the same way, even if some of the sources (like molasses) are more natural.

Most sugar sources have no vitamins or minerals and there are sixteen calories in one teaspoon of sugar. The average American conservatively consumes about twenty-two teaspoons of sugar a day, which equates to about 350 calories. Most of that sugar is hidden in packaged convenience foods. You might be surprised by some of the products that contain sugar, such as salad dressings or tomato sauces. Even some brands of bread have added sugar!

Sugar's addictive qualities adapt our taste buds to high sweetness, to the point where a fresh piece of fruit seems bland. Compared with high fiber foods that are filling and satisfying, sugary foods tend to be high in excess calories and low in satiating properties. So, we end up eating more while not staying full very long.

This doesn't mean you can't have desserts or sweet foods anymore. The key is to strategically utilize alternatives that provide some satisfying sweetness without huge amounts of sugar and calories. One of my strategies for satisfying my love for ice cream was to find a lower calorie frozen yogurt that provided a similar texture, but with half the calories and fat. Another strategy I've used is switching to dark chocolate. Dark chocolate has less sugar and more cacao than milk chocolate, and it's become my go-to.

There are also plenty of low-sugar versions of treats and several products that use monk fruit and/or stevia as sweeteners. Erythritol is another excellent low-calorie sweetener to try. But keep in mind, erythritol is a sugar alcohol, which can cause digestive issues in some people.

It is important to read your labels and look for better choices. Never choose food that lists sugar as one of the first three or four ingredients on the label. Many cereals, granola bars, and premade dishes have added sugar, so look for products that don't use added sweeteners. Do your homework when shopping. I prefer to research food choices online before heading to the grocery store, so I know exactly which products have no added sugar. If you plan, you won't need to stand in the aisles reading every label.

Practical Strategies for THE EXTRAS

1. Use spreads like hummus instead of dips like ranch.
2. Ask for dips, dressings, and sauces on the side at restaurants.
3. Look for lite or sugar-free versions of condiments.

4. Marinade meats and poultry with lite salad dressing like a lite balsamic vinaigrette or lite Italian dressing.
5. Dust parmesan cheese or nutritional yeast on veggies and meats when roasting and broiling for added flavor.
6. Choose dishes that don't need added condiments.
7. Avoid all foods that come prepared as fried, tempura, breaded, encrusted, or battered.
8. Avoid dishes with hollandaise, gravy, alfredo, glazes, and fondues.

Practical Strategies for REDUCING SUGAR

1. Swap regular jams for sugar-free jams (or try a homemade version using half the sugar).
2. Switch to sugar-free or low-sugar condiments like ketchup, dressings, or the syrups added to coffee drinks.
3. Bake with lakanto/monk fruit, Truvia or Swerve.
4. Switch to sugar-free gum, hard candies, and throat lozenges.
5. Substitute mashed banana or unsweetened applesauce in place of both sugar and oil when baking muffins and quick breads from scratch.
6. Use Medjool dates, which have a naturally potent sweetness, in home-baked foods. Mash the dates using a blender or food processor.
7. Keep a bottle of Stevia in your purse or bag to have with coffee or tea at restaurants.
8. Avoid cereals or yogurts with added sugar.
9. Try lower calorie versions of some of your favorite sweets, like swapping frozen yogurt for ice cream or choosing dark chocolate over milk chocolate.

PART III
Movement, Rest, and Progress Strategies

STRATEGY 12
Sleep

A good laugh and a long sleep
are the best cures in the doctor's book.
Irish Proverb

Sleep as a strategy can seem a bit cliché. Everyone knows how important sleep is, but understanding *how* it affects our weight and *why* it is so impactful could make the difference in your motivation to prioritize sleep.

Aside from the obvious effects of sleep deprivation such as cognitive impairment and fatigue, there is significant research that links chronic lack of sleep with obesity. It's not, however, simply an issue of the lack of enough hours. It's also about getting *good quality* sleep.

There are two key hormones related to the sleep-appetite cycle, called ghrelin and leptin. Ghrelin tells your body it's hungry and leptin tells your body when it's full or satisfied. When you are low on sleep, you have more ghrelin and less leptin running through your bloodstream. It's as simple as that. A lack of sleep has hormonal implications that lead to overeating. I've experienced this on days when I'm short on sleep and felt as if my appetite was insatiable. No amount of dedication and willpower can overcome the hormonal effects of sleep deprivation.

This is why I make sleep one of my most prioritized strategies. If you want to lose weight and maintain it over a lifetime, sleep is non-negotiable! One of your highest priorities should be going to bed and waking up at consistent times and making sure to leave yourself eight hours for a good night of rest, or more if you need it. However, it's not just about weight. Sleep deprivation can negatively affect your mental health, especially if you suffer from depression or anxiety.

I wish I could say that I've found a way to override a rise in a hormone like ghrelin or that willpower can get you through, but it's just not the case. Of course, there will be times when you can't help but run short on sleep. In that situation, you must give yourself a break because sometimes it is unavoidable. I have good luck when I rely on protein snacks to help with that extra strong hunger that I get when I'm sleep deprived. I also make a strong effort to get all my meals in on those days.

One male client that I worked with in the past was shocked to discover how effective this strategy was for him. He habitually stayed up late browsing the internet, claiming he just couldn't fall asleep on any kind of a schedule. He'd oversleep in the morning and wind up rolling out of bed, grabbing some coffee in a rush, and running off to work. In addition to causing havoc in his mornings, he set himself up to miss the workouts he had planned, and he often binged at lunch.

He became frustrated with our sessions when I refused to write out a diet for him. He was convinced that if I would just write a diet for him to follow each day, he could use that to bypass healthy habits. When I refused, he finally agreed to a fourteen-day "sleep challenge." He committed to going to bed at a set time while abstaining from TV and electronics. We established an acceptable ritual for him, which included a hot shower and reading a book of his choice for no more than thirty minutes. He set his alarm to wake up at the same time each morning.

At the end of the two weeks, this client came to me with an embarrassed smile as he admitted that my sleep strategy was exactly what he needed. He explained that after a few nights adjusting to his new routine, he woke up feeling refreshed and motivated. He had time for breakfast and, on some days, he had time to make lunch to bring to work.

Once he recognized the positive impacts of prioritizing sleep, I made a few more suggestions, including blackout curtains, to further enhance the quality of his sleep so he could truly maximize his health. He even began to ride his bike to work since he felt so much better in the morning.

This client was a great example of the ripple effects of good sleep habits. It is a foundational strategy without which everything else suffers.

Practical Strategies for SLEEP

1. Install blackout curtains or shades in your bedroom, because even small amounts of light can inhibit melatonin production. Melatonin is the body's sleep hormone that, when released, helps us fall asleep. The darker your room, the better. I would even suggest not keeping television sets or digital clocks in your bedroom to avoid even the tiniest sources of light.

2. Set the thermostat at the right temperature for sleep. A drop in core body temperature helps the body get into sleep mode, so cooling down the room is essential. Research suggests that sixty-eight degrees is, on average, a good place to set the thermostat for sleep. But you may find that you need it a little higher or lower than that based on whether you wake up too hot or cold in the middle of the night.

3. Invest in a comfortable bed and pillows for the best sleep quality. A good mattress can also help with some of your body's aches and pains. So, if you're already in the market for a new bed, now is a great time to start your search.
4. Consider sound machines and sleep sound apps. Random sounds from inside and outside your home can disturb REM sleep. So, having "white noise" consistently playing can prevent that disruption and sudden waking. Steady, uninterrupted sounds have been proven to help people sleep better and longer.
5. Limit your caffeine intake in the afternoon, especially if you have an early bedtime. I stop caffeine intake by 2:00 p.m. each day, but you might need to stop all caffeine-containing products (including chocolate) even earlier. Everyone metabolizes caffeine differently and it's useful to experiment to see how your sleep is affected by various cut-off times.
6. Be consistent with the time you go to bed each night. Research has shown that when you stick with a sleep schedule, going to bed and waking at the same time, you can improve overall quality of sleep and your ability to fall asleep.
7. Experiment with magnesium supplements taken at bedtime to help with sleep. Check with your personal physician to decide whether that might be a good option for you.

STRATEGY 13
The NEAT Strategy

One of the most important principles of success is developing the habit of going the extra mile.
Napoleon Hill

What is NEAT and how does it factor into the strategies? NEAT is an acronym that stands for Non-Exercise Activity Thermogenesis. What it refers to is basically all the activities of daily living outside of exercise.

I have my own story of how I developed respect for this important component of health and fitness because I never previously gave it much consideration.

I was at a point in my life when I felt like I'd really mastered weight management and exercise. I had maintained a healthy weight for decades and I was a dedicated daily exerciser. I put a lot of effort into my workouts and felt confident that I was pushing hard and giving a lot of energy to my fitness plan. I also felt like my diet was dialed in and consistent, but I noticed that I had gained some weight, and it was challenging to make any progress in getting back to my previous weight. My clothes were feeling tight, and I was frustrated and a bit confused.

So, I made sure to be careful of overt snacking and mindless eating. But I still hadn't bounced back. Then I realized something I wasn't considering. There was a change in my daily routine. I had lost my dog of sixteen years and realized that for her entire life, I'd been taking her for hikes on the weekends and regular walks during the week in addition to my own workouts. I realized I had a NEAT issue. I was sitting around a lot more and not going out for activity with my dog.

Even though I never counted the dog walks as "exercise" I knew it was the one thing in my life that had changed. I had taken those walks for granted, not really understanding how important they were for *both* of us. I began to have a newfound respect for NEAT and the powerful effects of daily activity. The extra movement we make can have a big impact on our overall health.

So, one of the first things I did was purchase a pedometer. I needed to see where my starting point was. How many steps I took on average showed me objectively how active or sedentary I was. I discovered I didn't move as much as I thought, and the scale told me that my workouts didn't afford me the luxury of sitting on my butt all day, which apparently I was doing. I kept the pedometer on for two weeks and tracked my daily average to get a baseline. Once I had my average, I made it my goal to do two thousand more steps than that baseline each day.

If I noticed my step count was low, I'd get up and do something. Sometimes, I cleaned the house, other times I went out and did the grocery shopping or other errands. I made sure to use the stairs whenever they were available and I parked my car a bit farther from the store, so I had to walk. If I was working at my desk, I made sure I got up and walked around frequently.

After increasing my steps by an additional two thousand, I upped the ante a bit more and got into a routine of averaging six thousand to eight thousand steps a day, which was enough to see changes without being too difficult to attain. It was a great learning experience and truly eye opening for me.

I eventually adopted two dogs who keep me busy, whether it's a walk, a hike, or an obedience class. Sometimes I just play with them in the backyard, but I'm so much more aware of my daily movement now. Even though NEAT isn't the same as hard exercise, it matters a great deal. NEAT is the missing element in so many people's lives. You might be putting in an effort and eating healthy yet can't figure out why you're stuck. Of course, there might be other things that need adjusting and improving, but NEAT is often overlooked.

It's deceptive because we don't think of cleaning the house as part of our plan for better health, but movement throughout the day is essential. It's an excellent, healthy habit to get out into the fresh air and sunshine and clear your mind while taking a walk. I promise, it improves your life on more levels than what's reflected on the scale.

If you're challenged by sitting at a desk all day at work, ask your employer if you could get an adjustable standing desk. Standing desks allow you to alternate between sitting and standing while working, and yes, standing counts as NEAT. It's healthier than sitting and better for your posture.

You also don't have to limit your NEAT to walks. Take your kids to the park or walk through a museum or aquarium. Look for classes to take with your pet where you get up and work with them. If the weather is bad, take care of an organizational project and clean out your closets or garage. There are so many options depending on your own situation of time, budget, and what activities you like to do, but if you're moving, it's NEAT and it's helping you get healthy.

If you can afford a pedometer, I strongly suggest you get one and wear it every day. The feedback you get, seeing your steps for the day, is invaluable. Quickly, you'll become aware of hidden opportunities for movement. For example, if you're in the airport all day and you have time before you board your flight, don't just sit and wait, do some laps around the terminal. Walk around and browse the stores.

If you need motivation to take walks, bring earbuds and listen to a podcast or audio books. Make it as enjoyable as you can and don't bring your work with you. Make it so that you look forward to it. When you clean the house, put on good music that you love so it doesn't feel like a chore. Make movement feel good so you'll want to do more of it.

Dedicated exercise is amazingly healthy for your body and mind, but it's not the whole picture when it comes to health and fitness. You need to be active throughout the day and take every opportunity to get up and move. Get creative and be consistent and you will find yourself naturally getting into the habit of utilizing NEAT.

Practical Strategies to BOOST NEAT

1. Park further away from stores in the parking lot as a habit.
2. Walk or bike to stores whenever the opportunity allows for it.
3. Take the stairs whenever they are available.
4. Wear a pedometer daily and track your steps, and set goals to increase your daily steps.
5. Utilize a standing/adjustable desk for work to get up on your feet as much as possible during the workday.
6. Make it a daily ritual to go out for walks with your pets or kids. Go to the park or bike together.
7. Incorporate activities when making travel plans. Find sightseeing that requires walking or biking through scenic areas.
8. Make a list of activities you can do when you need to boost your daily steps, like house cleaning, organizational projects, yard work, etc.

STRATEGY 14
Exercise

What seems impossible today
will one day become your warmup.
Unknown

Exercise is a well-known component of good health, but it's essential to understand the role of exercise and how it factors into weight loss and lifestyle. There is a huge misunderstanding with regards to exercise. While it *is* necessary for meeting your fitness goals, the misunderstanding is that exercise is the primary driver of weight loss. Most people think that if they just find the right class or get going on a new program, they'll start to automatically lose weight. This needs clarification. There are two well-known sayings in the fitness world: "You can't out-exercise a bad diet" and "abs are made in the kitchen." The point being made is that your diet is the most important factor in weight management. Exercise is just an *enhancement.*

I've had many clients who relied too heavily on exercise while continuing to struggle in pursuit of their goals. One in particular was a young female client of mine who was incredibly fit. She ran every morning before work, then she took fitness classes or lifted weights in the evenings. She was strong and athletic, but she couldn't understand why she wasn't reaching her goals.

When I looked at her food journal, I could see a lot of inconsistencies. Some days, it seemed she was eating too little for the amount of exercise she was doing, yet on other days, she was eating far more than she likely needed to meet her needs. When I spoke with her, she described her eating as "out of control." She admitted to bingeing on snacks and chips, but then "held it together" on the other days. I could see that she desperately needed to regain balance in her overall program.

When I asked her to drop from two exercise sessions per day down to one, she looked anxious, but I asked her to trust the process and I helped her see that what she was doing would be unsustainable. I emphasized the need for rest and recovery, and I explained that one strong effort per day was more than enough.

It took several weeks for her to adjust to fewer workouts, but once we brought her exercise into balance and focused on healthy meals with plenty of protein and fiber, she stopped binging on snacks and her body began to feel stronger since she was getting the appropriate rest she needed. Her appetite was also no longer in overdrive. It wasn't long before she started to see real progress, and best of all, she felt much better.

Relying too heavily on exercise can have other unintended consequences. For instance, I had a friend call me once, somewhat despondent. She was training for a marathon, which meant she was logging many miles of running each week. She was really confused and disappointed that she wasn't losing weight. I knew immediately what was going on. Heavy exercise can have a major effect on appetite. Your body needs a lot of calories when you're training intensely week to week. Her body kicked up its appetite to meet the demands of her marathon training. So, even though she was doing something healthy for her body by improving her cardiovascular conditioning, her body's caloric needs were dramatically rising as well. Therefore, she ate a lot more food each day to meet her body's demands.

I encouraged my friend to place her focus for the time being on fueling her body, staying strong, and following through on her marathon. Then, once she achieved her goal, we could look at her diet and shift back to weight management strategies, but it was important that she did not try to do both at the same time.

I don't want to discourage anyone from challenging their body with demanding fitness goals like running a marathon. It's amazing when someone takes on a big goal. I'm also not saying that there aren't great health benefits to that type of training. I'm merely pointing out that exercise shouldn't be used to compensate for poor food choices. There needs to be a balance of meeting your body's needs with healthy, nutritious foods, all while not *over-exercising* as a tool for weight loss. This is not the way to effectively use exercise and training programs. Not to mention that if you over-train, it can be rough on your joints and muscles if you haven't adapted to that level of fitness.

Exercise can enhance weight loss in addition to having many other health benefits. It can be excellent for your blood pressure, it can build bone density, and there is evidence to suggest that it can improve depression and anxiety, but it should not be used as the primary driver of weight loss. Exercise will enhance your weight loss efforts, but without sensible nutrition, it can only get you so far.

So, what is the best type of exercise and how much should you be doing each week? I've been asked many times, for example, if weight training or cardio is better for aiding weight loss. My answer is always the same…whichever type of exercise is most enjoyable for you is the best choice, because if you enjoy it, you're more likely to be consistent over a long period of time.

I personally like to mix things up and do a combination of resistance training, do a day or two each week of cardiovascular work for heart health, and go out for walks as active recovery. I might even add in a yoga class. Avoiding monotony is very important for me and I've discovered that variety helps keep me enthusiastic and motivated. You might prefer more consistency. You have to find out what works best for you.

If you are completely new to exercise, I recommend trying new things until you find something you love. There's no magic exercise other than the one you can stick with long-term.

You should plan your workout times and days for the week in advance. Never leave your exercise to chance. You should know the night before exactly what activity you'll do the next day, as well as the start time. Don't tell yourself that you'll decide what to do in the morning. It's too easy to get distracted with other home and work obligations.

Deciding how often to exercise should be part of your weekly planning and included in your schedule the same way you do so for an appointment. There can be some flexibility in the sense that you might have to work around your job or your kid's school schedule. Make exercise work with your personal situation. Just don't use life's obligations as an excuse for not training and taking care of yourself. Be honest about what is feasible and stick with it.

I believe for weight loss, four days a week is a good minimum goal, and if you do something rigorous for thirty to sixty minutes each time, then that's an excellent place to start.

Practical Strategies for EXERCISE

1. Plan your weekly exercise in advance so that you know exactly what to do each day.
2. Schedule your exercise on your calendar (with a start time) just like an appointment.
3. Choose one new class each week to try out until you find something you enjoy that feels sustainable.
4. Maintain your current exercise plan if you overindulge, and don't add more exercise to compensate for poor diet choices. Over-exercising will lead to burnout.
5. Consider hiring a trainer (if only for a limited time) so you can cultivate the habit of commitment and benefit from professional instruction.
6. Consider a subscription service for home workouts. The investment will help you stay accountable. Choose your classes for the week and plan a scheduled start time.
7. Find a workout buddy who you can depend on. But, if they continuously cancel on you or become a negative influence (because they goof off, for example), then cut them loose. A good workout buddy pushes you and shows up regularly on-time!

STRATEGY 15
Weighing Progress

It's not what we do once in a while that shapes our lives.
It's what we do consistently.
Anthony Robbins

Keeping track of your bodyweight has become a controversial topic over the years. The scale is sometimes perceived as a tool of self-shaming and there has been a negative association with attaching self-worth to a specific number (either your current bodyweight or your goal weight). It's unfortunate, because tracking your weight can be one of the most effective tools you have in order to clearly see progress. It's one way to know if what you're doing works or not, or if you need to adjust.

It's important to understand that I'm not suggesting you obsess over numbers. Tracking your weight should not become an unhealthy focus. In most cases, you can avoid weight-obsession by utilizing some guidelines combined with a bit of understanding about weight fluctuations.

First, I do not recommend weighing yourself more than twice a week. I use the scale once a week and that works well for me. Weighing more frequently leads to problematic issues. It's also not very effective to get on the scale too frequently because it's common to see fluctuations from day to day that often just reflect water retention, which is nothing to worry about. You might have a high-sodium meal one day, and as a result, the scale goes up several pounds the following morning. This is no cause for panic since water retention resolves on its own within a day or two.

Use the scale to see an overall, long-term trend, not a week-to-week drop in weight. You're looking for a month-to-month trajectory. You can log your weight in your day planner or phone to keep a clear picture of the direction you're headed as a reference. Then, adjust your plan as needed.

This will keep you accountable to your own goals. When things aren't moving in the right direction, assess your habits and be honest with yourself about slip ups, weekend alcohol and food binges, or your commitment to exercise. Keeping track of your numbers helps you stay aware of the choices you make.

When I graduated from college as a young twenty-something, I moved to Florida to start my career as a nutrition counselor and personal trainer. I had little experience working with others. But I had been training on my own for seven years at that point and I was armed with a degree in Dietetics. I was incredibly enthusiastic about educating my clients on all things diet and exercise.

I became disappointed, however, when I noticed a theme developing with my clientele. I felt like I was more motivated to see them succeed than they were. I began to observe that at the beginning of each week, my clients routinely joked about the dessert they had over the weekend or their big night of drinking. They were almost bragging about their indifference to the program I created for them.

I reached out to one of the other very successful trainers I worked with and told him what was happening, seeking his advice. He looked at me plainly and said that he fired clients like that. I was in complete shock. He laughed at the exasperated look on my face then explained that almost one hundred percent of the time the clients he fired begged him not to cut them loose and then, subsequently, they would do a complete 180 degree turn around and get back on track.

After giving his story much thought, I realized that my colleague's bold approach was like an ice-cold bucket of water over his client's heads. It was accountability slapping them across the face and it forced them to decide whether they truly wanted to quit or get serious.

I, on the other hand, had abdicated my duty to hold *my* clients accountable. They weren't lazy people, they were just giving in to human nature. Our brains are wired to avoid pain and seek comfort, and if I wasn't holding them accountable, then who was? Wasn't that what they had *really* hired me for? I hadn't been requiring my clients to do weekly weigh-ins or body measurements because I didn't want to upset them or make them feel bad. In actuality, I wasn't providing the structure or the tools to measure their progress or their commitment. That's one of the things a scale provides. It is not the *only* barometer of your success; it is a valuable tool that provides useful data to help you know what might or might not be working.

The feedback my coworker gave about his approach with clients was a valuable lesson I will never forget. From that moment on, you can believe that I instituted mandatory weekly check-ins, utilized a scale and measuring tape, and began to chart my clients' progress so that we could both clearly visualize whether they were moving towards their goals or not. I cannot overstate the effectiveness of this approach.

Like it or not (and most of us don't), weighing yourself on a scale each week is sometimes the only way to stay truly accountable to ourselves. Yes, you can also go by how your clothes fit and feel. Yes, you can also use a tape measure or a Dexa scan when one's available, but you must gauge your own progress and get real about your commitment.

Practical Strategies for WEIGHING PROGRESS

1. Purchase a high-quality scale and store it in a space where you can easily see it and access it.
2. Choose which day of the week you weigh yourself to gauge your progress. Be consistent and record your results.
3. Weigh yourself at the same time of day with preferably no clothes on. I believe the best time is immediately after getting out of bed in the morning.
4. Review your recorded numbers once a month to track progress and ensure that you see the trend going in the right direction.
5. Take photos of yourself each month as an additional progress tool (front, back, and side poses) in minimal clothing to monitor body composition changes.
6. Consider hiring a trainer to meet up with once a week to take measurements or to do your weigh-in. You have a greater chance of success with personal accountability.

STRATEGY 16
Macros, Prepping, and Tracking

A goal without a plan is just a wish.
Antoine de Saint-Exupery

Now that I've covered many of the basic strategies, it's time to pull everything together so you have concrete guidelines to work within. Refer now to the numbers you calculated and recorded in your notebook. Find the number you got using the Harris Benedict Equation. That number gives you a place from which to start and later adjust as needed. Remember that this equation is just an *estimate* of the base level of calories your body needs to maintain your current weight.

The easiest way to track your caloric intake is to use a macro-tracking app. There are many available to download for free, and if you find one you really love, you can typically upgrade to a fancier (paid) option down the road if you choose. However, I think the best way to start is to simply track the foods you eat to see where you're currently at. One of the nice features on many macro apps is that the app remembers foods once you've entered them. That means you don't have to keep searching for the same foods you eat regularly.

Use the macro tracker for about one week so you get used to the app and get an idea of how many calories you *currently* eat. Once you log a week's worth of food, you get a clearer picture of your habits, as well as your average calories, protein, fat, etc.

Once you've completed the first week, you have a rough idea of what it takes to *maintain* your weight. Now you can use this information to determine how much of a caloric deficit you need to drop your weight. Typically, it's best not to reduce calories by more than ten to twenty percent. For example, if you discover that you currently eat, on average, 2,500 calories per day, start with a minimum deficit of ten percent. That means you would set your caloric goal at 2,250 calories, reducing your daily intake by 250 calories.

The other way to approach this is to use the Harris Benedict Equation you calculated to determine your base number of calories and use that number as your next week's goal. Either way, it requires some trial and error to determine what your level of calorie intake has been. My recommendation, however, is to try and get the most results from the least reduction in calories, because *there is no sense in reducing more than it takes to get a result.* It is best to aim to keep the highest calories possible while still losing weight. Extremes are not only unnecessary, but they are also detrimental, unsustainable, and quickly lead to binging.

Calories are only one aspect of tracking. Macronutrients or "macros" refer to the nutrients your body needs for basic health and wellness, including protein, carbohydrates, and fat. Just for comparison, micronutrients are the vitamins and minerals your body needs in trace amounts to sustain healthy function. It is easiest for beginners to focus primarily on total calories and protein. Carbohydrates and fats are neither good nor bad, and neither should be restricted or avoided. Rather, I believe it is a better approach to focus on protein and eat carbs and fats according to your palate and preference. You should, however, take care not to let your fat go below 0.3 grams per pound of body weight, as this would be the bare minimum necessary for optimal health. Dietary fat is healthy and necessary in reasonable amounts.

As I mentioned in the protein strategy, protein is very satiating. Eating protein-rich foods will increase your success. As a bonus, adequate protein helps preserve lean muscle tissue, which is especially important since muscle tissue burns calories and increases basal metabolic rate. So, a good rule of thumb is to set your protein goal between 0.8 grams and 1.0 gram per pound of bodyweight. This is a common recommendation that is very effective at preserving lean tissue.

If I have a client who is a 165-pound female currently eating 2,500 calories as her baseline, I will start with a ten percent calorie deficit equaling 2,250 calories per day. If her goal weight is 140 pounds and I'm aiming for 1.0 gram of protein per pound of bodyweight, she would set her calorie goal on her tracker to 2,250 calories, with 140 grams of protein per day.

The best way to make it easy for her to meet her protein goals is to decide how many meals she wants to eat each day and divide her protein by that number. So, if she decided that she could eat four meals a day (breakfast, lunch, dinner, and snack) then she would plan approximately forty-one grams of protein in *each* of those four meals.

It initially takes some work to learn the amount of protein in foods, but the macro tracker apps can help you with that as well, because as you record food, you see how many grams of protein are in a serving. If you need more, then increase your serving sizes accordingly.

Tracking calories and macros gets easier with time. I spend a minute, tops, on entering my data, and it also allows me to track whatever nutrients I want to pay attention to, including fiber, sugar, sodium, etc.

I've walked many people through this process. What's been most rewarding is seeing how tracking has empowered them to make simple adjustments on their own. Many of them gained the confidence to make informed decisions about their food choices because they had greater awareness about what they were eating each day.

Meal Prep

Preparing your food for the week in advance is the next critical step in hitting your goals. Prep makes life so much easier, and it ensures that you are never without the food you need to make the best choices. Start by picking a day each week when you plan to do all your grocery shopping and food preparation. I've included a sample grocery list in the back of this book to use as a guideline for shopping. As you progress, you can adjust this list to suit your tastes and preferences.

Once you get home with your groceries, remove all the produce from containers and bags, and wash everything right away. Put fresh fruit out in bowls, and then chop and store your vegetables. From that point, you can either cook up protein and veggie batches (which is the best approach) or keep everything cut and ready to cook in the refrigerator.

If you choose to cook everything, make big batches such as baked chicken breasts, grilled bison, and lean ground turkey burgers, etc. Then, after everything has cooled, package it all up in containers so it's ready to grab and go during the week. You can also experiment with batches of soup in the slow cooker, roasted vegetables, and any healthy homemade goods you want to have on hand. Hardboiled eggs are also excellent to keep in the refrigerator for busy days.

Other great foods that do well in big batches are low-fat cabbage slaws, pre-cooked spaghetti squash that can be re-heated with tomato sauce for a veggie-based spaghetti, or a sloppy joe mix made with equal parts lean ground beef and lean ground turkey. If you're willing to do the research, find healthy food bloggers who specialize in low-sugar, high protein meals.

Keep healthy fats in your pantry to add to your meals in small quantities. Fat sources to avoid include fats from processed vegetable oils, fried foods, margarine, and shortening, but some of the healthy fats are as follows:

- Olive oil
- Avocado
- Coconut oil
- Real butter and ghee (clarified butter)

Other sources of healthy fats:

- Fatty fish like salmon
- Nuts and nut butters like almond, cashew, and walnut butter (in limited amounts)
- Seeds such as pumpkin and sunflower seeds
- Whole eggs (the yolk contains fat)
- Dark chocolate

Keeping avocados on hand to add to meals is a great idea, but they go bad quickly. I store either a bag of frozen avocado chunks in the freezer or I buy mini guacamole packs to use as a spread. Nut butters are very concentrated in calories, so I prefer to purchase nut butter *packets,* which come in a sealed serving size.

When I purchase nuts and seeds, I weigh and portion out one-ounce baggies in advance so that I have a grab-and-go snack. Pre-measured snacks like this are handy, and in a time-crunch, they provide excellent nutrition without ruining your food plan for the day.

For quick carbohydrate sources, I have my (gluten-free) breads and English muffins on hand in the freezer, so they keep for a long time and can be re-heated quickly in a toaster. Rice cakes keep for a long time as well, and when I crave something crunchy, I spread them with hummus. While unprocessed whole foods are ideal, it's important to have a variety of choices available.

The more you prepare, stock up, and cook each week, the greater your chances for success. Always set aside time in your calendar for grocery shopping and food prep. Then, re-stock your purse, workbag, and car with healthy snacks for the week. This prepares you for any traffic jam, weather delay, or unexpected crisis you might encounter. You'll stay on track, but you'll be less stressed when obstacles show up in your path.

Practical Strategies for MACROS, PREPPING, AND TRACKING

1. Store your grocery list on your phone so that you always have it when you need it.
2. Find a macro tracker you like that is easy for you to use. I prefer "My Net Diary," but there are multiple options.
3. Look for healthy recipes you can make in large batches, then store your prepared food in the refrigerator or freezer so that you always have good meals when you're short on time.
4. Store foods in the freezer that are great for quick grabs. Gluten-free or whole-grain breads (light versions) can

easily be defrosted and toasted. Store bananas, avocado chunks, and berries in the freezer for smoothies.

5. Purchase organizer bins for the refrigerator and pantry to keep your food organized and easy to find.
6. Try a meal delivery service that caters to healthy eaters so that you always have a healthy choice to pull out of the freezer and re-heat for days when you're too tired to make something.
7. Use single serving nut-butter packets.

PART IV
Mindset Strategies

STRATEGY 17
Visualizing Your Success

You can't do anything that you can't picture yourself doing.
Anonymous

How you start your day has a tremendous impact on how your day unfolds. It can influence your attitude and have a huge impact on your mood. Morning rituals are more important than most people realize. Starting every single day with ten minutes of meditation and visualization can have powerful cumulative effects on your ability to succeed in reaching your goals.

Visualization has been used successfully by professional athletes, performance artists, musicians, and public speakers for decades. Research has shown measurable effects on physical performance through the utilization of visualization techniques. When you practice visualization, your brain doesn't know the difference between the physical act of what you are imagining versus the mental and emotional state of imagining it.

The key to effective visualization is to connect the detailed images in your mind to the emotions you would feel having achieved what you envision. For example, if you see yourself in your mind's eye looking fit and healthy, you want to simultaneously conjure the feelings of the joy and freedom that you'd experience having achieved your goal. You can also use your imagination to envision yourself getting your daily exercise done and going through your day making healthy choices, but you need to link those images with the positive emotions.

Challenging goals *must* feel attainable to motivate you each day to follow through on your plans. Visualization is a simple, effective tool that enables you to cultivate a sense of what is truly possible. It is *essential* to nurture your dreams and the feel-good emotions that connect you directly to your aspirations. Journaling is another way to further cement your resolve after you visualize. Make a list of affirmations that support your success and read them through each morning after your meditation.

The other benefit to starting your day with visualization is that it gives you a brief period of *time-out* at the beginning of the day to make an active choice about how you want your day to unfold. Use that time to set an intention to meet your personal goals for the day. Consistent, daily visualization can strengthen your resolve in such a powerful way that it eventually affects your behavior and choices in productive ways.

Your own mind can be your greatest ally…
so use it for your own benefit!

In the past, when I've asked clients to incorporate visualization into their morning ritual, I've seen my share of eye rolls. Some have expressed frustration that I've asked them to include something that seems insignificant compared with other lifestyle changes that I've asked them to work on. One client, who was a woman in midlife, struggling through a tough divorce and significant weight gain from the stress, literally said to me "you've got to be kidding!"

She went on to protest that she had way too much to deal with, emotionally and physically, to worry about the "silly meditation" I was asking her to do. She was exasperated by all the change and didn't understand how visualization would help her.

However, I knew it was *precisely* what she needed. So, instead of explaining how this tool could be helpful, I decided to guide her through a brief visualization as part of our weekly check-ins. I began each session with a ten-minute guided meditation.

After using this approach only two times, she told me that she had begun to incorporate the practice a few times a week on her own, recreating the guided sessions we had done together in my office. She told me that our office sessions helped her relax after her long days and that she noticed she left feeling better. It inspired her to try them at home.

This tool affected my client's entire attitude. She acknowledged that the daily visualization provided the one chance she had each day to relax and focus on *her* needs and goals. It helped her organize her thoughts and envision her progress in a way she had never done previously. She felt more motivated and prepared for whatever the day might bring. Additionally, as her coach, I noticed a positive change in her entire approach. She went from dreading the changes to seeing them as the path to achieve her deep desire to regain her health.

By taking the time every morning to cultivate a strong image of what you choose to accomplish, you reinforce your confidence that you *can* reach your goals. You also begin to cultivate a healthier inner dialogue. That emerging confidence translates into changes in your attitude and decisions.

Don't overcomplicate it. Just sit, relax, and use your imagination to place the focus on your dreams. Once you have the images in your mind, allow yourself to feel the emotions of achievement. In other words, don't imagine what *could* be possible in the future…rather, see yourself having already attained success and imagine how it *feels* having already reached your goals. That's the key to this practice. Know what it feels like and experience your success.

I prefer to keep my practice limited to ten minutes because it feels sustainable. Find the timeframe that works for you. If you find yourself getting restless or impatient, then stop. Keep it enjoyable and easy to manage as a daily practice.

Practical Strategies for VISUALIZATION

1. Reserve a space for yourself where you can get at least ten minutes of quiet, uninterrupted time. This might require that you set your alarm to be up before everyone else. Or you could choose a room where everyone in your home knows not to enter when the door is closed in the morning.
2. Ensure that you leave yourself enough time that you don't feel pressured or rushed so you can completely relax and get focused.
3. Try noise-canceling headphones or some inexpensive ear plugs. The more you can shut out distractions, the more effective your practice will be.
4. Experiment with different timers. A meditation app with a timer or a watch alarm will do. If you set a timer for ten or fifteen minutes (depending on how much time you want to take), it eliminates the need to keep looking at the clock.
5. Use ten deep, relaxing breaths to settle in before starting the visualization process, so that you ready yourself to focus completely.

6. Create a comfortable space to sit and keep the lights low. You can pick a chair or even sit up in bed. Try to avoid lying flat, as it tends to lead to falling asleep. You want to stay alert but relaxed.
7. Review how your day went at bedtime and take a moment to feel gratitude for all the positive choices you made, or write out a gratitude list to acknowledge your successes, however big or small.

STRATEGY 18
Feeding your Mind

The happiness of your life
depends upon the quality of your thoughts...
Marcus Aurelius

Consider that we are all a product of our environment. The space you live in, the shows you watch, the people you hang out with. They all play an important role in the choices you make and how you feel. For example, your home can either be an uplifting and supportive space, or it could, potentially, bring you down. Don't underestimate the impact your state of mind has on even small, everyday choices. A positive mindset can mean the difference between sitting down on the couch to watch TV for four hours versus going for a walk and getting fresh air and exercise. If you feel good, you generally feel more energized and motivated to make good choices.

This applies not only to your home, but also where you work plus what and who you expose yourself to on a regular basis. If you have friends who try to sabotage your efforts, it might be worth reconsidering how much time you spend with them. Surround yourself with people who support you.

The same goes for your work environment. You might spend eight hours or more a day at work. If work is filled with negative colleagues and bad attitudes, you can be sure it rubs off on you whether you recognize it or not. Maybe you work in a space where you are literally exposed to toxic chemicals or poor air quality. It's something to consider. Of course, we all can't just up and quit, and I'm not suggesting that. You might, however, think about your options and whether you need to make new choices, if you are able to.

Give some thought to what you're reading. How does that material make you feel? What are you watching on TV? Does the news bring you down or give you anxiety? Stop watching it! Don't feed your mind anything that lowers your mood or gives you anxiety. Stop following social media pages that make you feel bad about yourself or cause you to compare yourself to others. Only follow content that *inspires* you. Clear out all the negative and use technology to serve *your* goals. It can be hard to let go of that stuff, but if you are truly committed to changing your habits, you must change your state of mind.

Look for new podcasts or audio books for your commute to work and pick interesting subjects that make your ride enjoyable. Choose movies and TV series that educate or inspire. Never waste your time on mental junk food that leaves you feeling worse. One of the reasons I stopped watching crime dramas a long time ago was because I experienced restless sleep or nightmares afterwards. I'll choose a comedy any day over a murder mystery.

If you've never made a vision board before, try it out. It's a great way to get focused on what you want to create in your life for the coming year. There are plenty of online guides to help you navigate how to get started with your board. It's all part of the process of setting yourself up for success, so that you continually cultivate a positive state of mind.

If you constantly cave to temptations of the unhealthy foods lying around your pantry, you're not going to feel very positive about your progress. This is why it is so important to clean out the kitchen and cupboards of unhealthy foods. It's also critical to have a clean, well-organized kitchen, which makes food prep easier, and impacts the choices you make. If lots of healthy options are available and easy to find in the front of your refrigerator, you are more likely to make the right choices. Wipe out the refrigerator once a week, throw out food that's gone bad, and make room for new groceries.

Whatever you can do to make your entire living space inviting and inspiring can go a long way towards lifting your spirits. Keep the house clean, add fresh flowers, play good music. It cannot be overstated how important these elements factor into your mindset, which is everything when you make big lifestyle changes.

I had a friend in college who was struggling with depression. She couldn't seem to shake herself out of the habit of making destructive choices. She was drinking heavily on the weekends, she was not getting her work done, and her grades were dismal. I recall meeting her at her house one day and I felt immediate concern when I walked into her bedroom. There were so many clothes on the floor that I couldn't move my feet. Empty dishes were scattered around, and the bed didn't look as if it had been made in a while. It was obvious why she couldn't make it to class on time.

Gratefully, she sought help and began meeting with a therapist weekly. After a few months, I noticed a huge improvement in her mood, and she looked healthier and happier. She loved her therapy sessions, and I asked what she had found most helpful. She told me that her therapist asked her to prioritize cleaning and organizing her room. I wondered how cleaning her room related to the other things going on in her life. It seemed a bit backwards to me for the counselor to start with a room cleaning. My friend relayed what her therapist emphasized to her: *Your living space is a direct reflection of what is going on in your mind.* Therefore, she directed my friend to put the necessary time and attention into her living environment and to notice how the changes affected her.

My friend told me that she immediately noticed a sense of relief and her anxiety started to ease. The act of organizing also gave her a very tangible activity to start with. She told me that completing the task gave her a sense of control over the direction of her life, which allowed her to begin to proactively make the other changes she felt she needed. It was sort of a reverse approach. Clearing her living space seemed to give her space to think more clearly.

Watching this situation unfold with my friend had a huge impact on how I looked at my own environment. I've never forgotten the words of her therapist and seeing, firsthand, how the simple act of changing her living space had such profound effects on her life and state of mind. I've since utilized this approach multiple times throughout my own life and I'm a true believer in its power. I love to clean out stagnant spaces in my house when I feel stuck in my life. It feels like I'm creating space for something new to come forward.

In addition to bringing benefit to your own life, you can also use this as an opportunity to be of service to others. As you clean and reorganize, consider donating items to a local charity. It feels amazing to donate anything you're no longer using to someone who really needs it. Include your closet in this process. Toss any clothing that doesn't bring out the best in you. You should feel good in your clothes regardless of your weight and size, because the more confident and positive you feel now, the more inspired you will be to stay on your new, healthy path.

Practical Strategies for MINDSET

1. De-clutter your house or living space and get rid of old magazines and books.
2. Organize your closet and donate the clothing you no longer wear.
3. Scan your social media accounts. Delete or unfollow any accounts that don't uplift you.
4. Search for podcasts and audio books that inspire you.
5. Cancel subscriptions that don't serve you on your new path.
6. Buy fresh flowers for your home and put them where you see them every day.
7. Stop watching news, movies, etc. that give you anxiety or interrupt your sleep.

STRATEGY 19
Distraction Strategies

Idle hands are the devil's playthings.
Proverb

The same concept in the proverb above applies to all areas of your life. This is especially true when you're actively trying to make a lifestyle change. It's normal to feel resistance to change, even if you desperately want the change to happen. That inner resistance tries to sabotage your well-intended efforts. There's only one way to work around that: don't allow yourself to be idle. When you're bored or tired or frustrated, or when you just feel like being lazy, that's when you're the most vulnerable to self-sabotage. Emotional upsets can also trigger binges that make you feel much worse in the long run.

Have a plan in place for those times when you are most at risk of going off track. If you have strategies ready, then you have the resources you need to get back on track. It's important to give a lot of thought to what works best for you *before* you are in trouble. I have lots of suggestions for you to try, but you need to put them into action and see what works best.

There's a spectrum of strategies that I like to use based on a given situation. Some daily habits that I utilize on a regular basis help with formally ending my meal. They help stop cravings, so I don't eat more than I planned.

Chewing gum or brushing your teeth after a meal stops cravings and signals to your brain the time for eating is over. I keep a brush kit with toothpaste in my purse because it stops my sugar cravings. I also use mouthwash for the same purpose. Putting food away when you're done is helpful, as well.

When you're at home, put leftovers in containers and get everything into the refrigerator at the end of a meal. When food is left in sight, you're much more likely to keep picking at it. This is one of the reasons baking can be tricky. I enjoy baking, for example, but while goodies cool on the counter, I have a hard time leaving them alone. For the same reason, I don't recommend keeping candy in jars on counters and tables. It is way too tempting!

Other activities I rely on when I feel vulnerable to snacking include cleaning the house (which is also great for getting extra movement) or going outside to walk the dogs. Scheduling a massage or another spa service you like is an excellent way to take care of yourself in a positive way while sticking to your plan. When you hang out with friends, make sure your time doesn't revolve around food. Look for different activities you can do with friends that involve physical activity like a farmer's market, a pumpkin patch, or walking through the park.

Make a list of places you want to check out and start going through the list. You'll likely discover new places in your town you weren't even aware of. Getting out of the house to see new things will help you associate activity with good feelings, and you won't want to sit inside any longer.

If you have an engagement to go to where you know there will be a lot of unhealthy, tempting food options, such as a wedding, or a work event, eat something small (but filling) beforehand. No one will know, but when you don't show up ravenous, you won't be tempted to gorge on the appetizers or bread bowl.

Having a plan in place for events helps, too. If you have a friend or partner attending the same event, ask them to be your back-up. When you feel like you have an ally who understands your struggles, you can ask them for support. They can be your dance partner at a party who helps you focus on fun rather than all the food.

The bottom line is that we all like to binge on goodies and we all go overboard from time to time. Whether it's boredom, self-sabotage, or anxiety doesn't matter. The end result usually doesn't feel too good. Creating distractions is a way to circumvent your bad habits. Willpower is not a magic power only certain lucky people have. You just need to cultivate the discipline of preparation with a little forethought.

Practical Strategies for DISTRACTION

1. Purchase a few travel-sized toothpastes and toothbrushes to keep in your purse or car.
2. Buy packs of your favorite sugar-free mints and gum to keep on hand.
3. Plan activities in advance for your days off so that you don't wind up sitting on the couch snacking all day.
4. Take naps when you need them. Napping is good self-care, and it is better to catch up on much needed sleep than to mindlessly snack.
5. Keep small, healthy snacks available to eat before events.

STRATEGY 20
The Missing Element

We are what we repeatedly do.
Excellence, then, is not an act, but a habit.
Will Durant

When all is said and done, and you put forth the effort to make the strategies work, but accountability is not actively engaged, then the chances of long-term success decrease exponentially. Rare is the individual who achieves every goal one hundred percent of the time without any help at all. You need support, encouragement, and help along the way, as you make your way towards your goals.

The best fitness competitors and athletes have a support system that helps guide them along the way. Professional athletes have teams of experts who manage their health, their workouts, and nutrition. Coaches, personal trainers, and nutritionists are valuable assets to anyone who wants to get into shape or become fit. But the most valuable component of having a coach or trainer isn't just their knowledge. They provide the missing element in your overall approach to weight loss and improved fitness: accountability!

When you have no accountability, your goals and aspirations become flexible and bend easily with every sideshow and obstacle that pops up in life. There will never be a perfect time to pursue your goals and there will never be a scenario in which no setbacks arise. There will always be temptations, emotionally challenging situations, stressful living circumstances, and pressing obligations to throw you off track.

However, when you have accountability, it instills a superpower in you. You cultivate a stronger resolve and greater resiliency. Answering to yourself, *as well as others*, is a powerful motivator. When you ask for help, you build a team of people who encourage you along the way. They lift you up when things get rough or when you experience setbacks.

The "Weighing Your Progress" strategy is the first step in becoming accountable. Measuring your progress each week is the most tangible way to receive direct feedback on your efforts, but sometimes that isn't enough.

When I was a personal trainer, I had many clients who came to me frustrated by their lack of progress. They were trying the best they could, but success eluded them. Some of my clients already knew how to work out. They caught on easily to the programs I designed for them, but the real changes happened when we met each week to troubleshoot nutrition and lifestyle issues. It would often become a bit of a confessional, to which I gave feedback. I included weigh-ins to ensure I was helping them reach their goals, and clients repeatedly told me that our meetings motivated them to stick with their plan.

Having another person who is completely objective is often the missing element. It is incredibly powerful to share your goals with someone who is monitoring your progress. Don't choose a family member or friend; it must be someone who can objectively give you constructive criticism. When you make a financial investment, you will be more serious about it.

While it is possible to use online coaching, there's no doubt that in-person meetings are the best and most effective. Meeting face to face allows you to build a relationship with your coach and makes your goals more personal to them.

Not everyone needs this strategy, but most people benefit from having a professional to whom they are accountable. You may see great results on your own for a time, but it's not uncommon to hit a plateau and lose momentum. I have personally gone years at a time where I managed to maintain my fitness just fine, but then I struggled and used a coach to get back on track. No matter how much experience I have, I can always learn something new from another coach.

There are always ways to work around budget restrictions or time constraints, but never let fear or hesitancy keep you stuck in a cycle of failure and regrets. Fear and embarrassment are the most common reasons that keep people from seeking out accountability coaches. There are many professionals who love helping others achieve their fitness and weight loss goals, and they are excellent resources. With a little creativity, you can find a way to work with a coach while simultaneously staying within your budget and scheduling constraints.

Practical Strategies for THE MISSING ELEMENT

1. Hire a personal trainer if only for a monthly check-in. Sit down with them and explain that you specifically need accountability and supportive solutions to any issues you experience. Face-to-face accountability is a powerful motivator.

2. Meet with a trainer two to four times a week (four is ideal if you can afford it), for both exercise instruction and progress check-ins.

3. Hire a nutrition coach if it's within your budget.

4. Set up phone or online accountability check-ins if necessary. Ask for progress photo check-ins. Find a way to gauge improvements or setbacks.
5. Look for online communities where members provide support and offer recipe ideas and their own successful strategies.
6. Consider therapeutic counseling if you feel like you need emotional support. It is not uncommon for those who struggle with health and weight issues to have underlying emotional struggles from childhood or a specific event that led to unhealthy habits. There is no shame in seeking emotional support and it should always be confidential. In this way, you hold your internal stressors accountable.

Conclusion

Now that you have the fundamental tools to begin your successful weight loss journey, I want to leave you with a few thoughts. Even the most motivated and well-intentioned individuals hit roadblocks. Your path will be no different. Don't be discouraged by this. If you're prepared, you will be empowered to manage whatever comes up. The strategies that I've presented work when implemented consistently. When you encounter setbacks, know that the next step is to get right back in the game. Pick up this book, re-read a chapter or maybe a few. Refresh your resolve and start fresh again right away. Expect obstacles and be ready for them by cultivating an attitude of resilience. The only defeat is the one you *resign* yourself to accepting.

Keeping that in mind, let me prepare you for some of the most common hurdles clients and many others have presented to me along the way. (I've experienced these too, by the way!)

HEALTHY FOOD DOESN'T TASTE GOOD

This is one of the most common complaints I've heard over the years. It's legitimate and it actually has several components to it. If you feel irritated because you're deprived of your favorite, rich foods, there is a psychological adjustment. Change is hard. It makes us grumpy, and you are not alone in this. You must remember *why* you choose to eat differently. This issue resolves itself if you continue to focus on your *why*. Use your mindset strategies!

The other primary aspect is that your taste buds require time to adapt. Taste buds literally need time to adapt to new flavors. When I was a kid at birthday parties, I would beg my friends for their frosting flowers from the top of the cake! I was so accustomed to super sweet foods I couldn't get enough of them. These days, frosting tastes way too sweet for me. Frosting is unappealing now because my taste buds have adjusted to a different way of eating. Give yourself time with this. You will start to crave healthy, fresh food and you'll enjoy the new flavors more and more after just a few weeks.

Finally, you need to do a little leg work. Try new recipes and different restaurants that focus on healthy options. You will begin to discover new foods and dishes you had no idea you'd love so much! There are a lot of amazing options once you know what you're looking for.

I AM HUNGRY ALL THE TIME

If you are accustomed to eating a high volume of food or you've been snacking continuously throughout the day, you will experience some hunger as you change your ways. You cannot eat all you want and lose weight without any discomfort. People who are overweight or obese often eat too much of the wrong foods. You won't feel hungry forever, but there is a reasonable adjustment period. I once had a coworker who was gravely overweight, and I watched him every afternoon at lunch time as he returned to the office with a twelve-inch sub from the local sandwich shop. He'd have a meatball and cheese sub along with a large fountain soda and a bag of chips. The quantity of food combined with the calorie density was enough for three meals. Had he swapped out that sandwich for a six-inch sub on whole grain bread and loaded it with vegetables and lean protein, it would have provided lots of filling fiber to create a satisfying meal. I would also swap the soda for a zero-calorie drink to save on hundreds of empty calories.

It's normal to have some hunger between meals, especially if you are used to a large quantity of food. The best strategies to focus on in this instance are the protein and fiber strategies. Make protein and fiber top priorities at every meal. Your appetite will recalibrate in a short time when you give it the chance.

I AM TIRED AND UNMOTIVATED

It is true that eventually, the healthier you eat, you will gain energy and feel more alert throughout your day. But there is a transition period in which you might feel worse. If you have been loading up on stimulants like caffeine and sugar in sodas and junk food, you might feel sluggish. You will feel better than you have ever felt before when you stick with healthy eating, but your body needs excellent care during the transition.

Sleep as much as your body needs to replenish and recover. Include daily naps if you need to. Hydrate throughout the day with pure water and electrolytes. Lethargy is one of the signs of dehydration. Also remember to never rely on motivation. If you wait around for it to suddenly appear in your life, you might spend your whole life waiting. Motivation is fickle. Discipline is the *real* key to making things happen, and the good news is that discipline is something *everyone* can cultivate over time. In fact, science backs this. There is an area of the brain called the anterior mid-cingulate cortex. It is the area of the brain related to will and the willingness to persevere. It develops and grows stronger when you challenge yourself to do difficult things. You have the power to grow your discipline!

I CHEATED AND NOW I FEEL LIKE A FAILURE

I guarantee you that every person who has ever tried to change their eating habits has given in to cravings. This is usually followed by self-doubt and disappointment. It's a normal and expected part of the process. The trap to watch out for is how your mind reacts to this diversion. You might want to give up and throw in the towel. Truthfully, though, you need to dig deep to find your determination by remembering the reason you chose to make a change in the first place. Once again, remember your WHY. One slip here and there does not define your ability to succeed or not. What will determine the ultimate outcome is whether you are able to get back in the saddle. Your very next meal is your opportunity to course correct. Continue with your plan to exercise. Guilt is self-defeating and it is useless to you. Kick it to the curb and get right back on your program with your *very next meal*!

I'VE BEEN MISSING EXERCISE

This is bound to happen. Life gets busy and things get in your way. A flat tire, your manager asking you to stay late, having a sick kid home from school. Any number of distractions will get in the way of your workout. You must have a back-up plan and never let more than a day or two go by without movement. For example, a common obstacle many people face is weather diversions. Let's say you're someone who enjoys walking, running, or biking outdoors and suddenly your state is hit by a snowstorm. Have a backup plan that works for you. That plan might include indoor equipment like a treadmill or stationary bike. It might also include a workout video that you use for those occasions so you can train indoors. This is also one of the reasons I choose to workout first thing in the morning, when there is a less likely chance something will get in the way of my exercise.

Make a plan and then a back-up to the plan. Think ahead about the potential obstacles that might prevent you from doing your daily exercise. Strategize for the days when everything falls apart. What will you do? What will be your work-around? Do you want to invest in bad weather gear or home equipment? Maybe find some at-home workout videos that you save just for days when all your plans fall apart. Worst case scenario when obstacles are insurmountable, get back on track the very next day.

I'M ON A VERY TIGHT BUDGET

First, I completely get it. There was a time in my life when I could not afford a gym membership or online subscriptions. I had no disposable income, but I had massive determination. So, instead of giving up, I found creative ways to work out on the cheap. I alternated days running and doing some old power yoga tapes (yes, they were VHS!). I did this for two years and I had practically memorized the yoga series and wore out those tapes! But I am so glad that I didn't let my challenging financial state get in the way of my goals and that I refused to use it as an excuse. When I was in school, I worked one day a week at the local gym checking people in at the front desk just so I could get the free membership. Now, there are so many free workouts online that it's just a matter of finding the ones you like. Don't worry about having fancy workout clothes, either. Some inexpensive sweatpants and a t-shirt are all you need for most indoor workouts.

I have a friend who has a side hustle washing windows. He uses his service to barter for his membership. Look for creative solutions. Use your skills to trade for coaching and training guidance. Power walking is one of the least expensive forms of exercise. Find a local school that has an outdoor track you can use. Search for free online workouts. The possibilities are endless!

I STOPPED SEEING PROGRESS

This is an obstacle I'm very familiar with. Whether you've been living a healthy lifestyle for many years, or you are completely new to this, plateaus happen. It's extremely common and sometimes you just need a re-boot. Take a hard look at what you're doing and why you're doing it. Honestly assess your macro tracking. Are you being accurate? Maybe, lately, you've been spending more time talking at the gym than working out. Get some earbuds and listen to music to help keep you focused, or switch to exercise classes where you have an instructor to keep you on track during class. You might have slipped into a rut. Review the strategies and be truthful about any area that needs renewed focus and attention. Check out new books and podcasts that are meant to inspire.

When I hit a slump, I like to go back to the principles of the preparation stage. I de-clutter my living space and clear out my refrigerator and pantry. For me, that process signals a reset. I feel like I'm making a fresh start. A good, sweaty workout is another great way for me to re-focus. Plateaus often signal that something needs to change. It can be your workout intensity, your N.E.A.T activities or too many diet slips. Reassess, make the necessary changes, and move forward.

Now it's time to start your new, healthier life. I am beyond grateful that you chose to pick up this book and read it through to the end, but this is just the beginning for you. I hope that you re-visit these strategies whenever you feel stuck, want to refresh your knowledge, or need to renew your commitment. I am confident these tools will work for you. They have never let me down over the thirty-plus years I've developed and used them myself.

For ongoing support, I invite you to visit my website, strategicweightlossbook.com, for lots of free tips, recipes, and inspiration. I hope this is the start of your most exciting and healthy chapter yet!

APPENDIX A
Emergency Food Ideas

Helpful Storage Ideas:

- Purchase a small, dedicated freezer (to keep in the garage or basement).
- Bring a small, portable cooler with you to work (or keep it in the car).
- Use your purse or laptop bag to store a few snacks.
- Purchase a shaker bottle to quickly mix protein shakes.
- Reuse water bottles for water and sugar-free drinks.
- Keep hot or cold liquids with insulated steel bottles (Hydro Flask is a favorite).
- Shop with insulated reusable grocery bags.
- Carry food in Ziplock bags.
- Choose glass Tupperware for food prep and storage.
- Utilize a food saver vacuum packaging system (for more effective long-term storage in the refrigerator or freezer).
- Keep wide-mouth glass mason jars on hand for easy storage.

Examples of portable snacks:

(GF = Gluten Free, DF = Dairy Free)

- Perfect Amino Bars, 220-240 calories / GF
- Rx Bars, 210 calories / GF
- Raw Revolution bar (Ex. Chunky Peanut Butter Chocolate), 200 calories / GF / DF / Vegan
- Vega One snack bar (Ex. Dark Chocolate Cashew), 200 calories / GF / DF / Vegan
- Kind bars (Ex. Cranberry Almond + Antioxidants), 190 calories / GF / DF
- Larabars (Ex. Blueberry Muffin), 190 calories / GF / DF / Vegan
- 1 large banana, 100 calories
- Fage 2% Greek yogurt, 120 calories
- 1 slice Food for Life Ezekiel toast (7 Sprouted Grains), 80 calories
    - with ¼ avocado smashed on top as a spread, 90 calories (total 170 calories)
- 1 ounce raw nuts (almonds), 170 calories
- 1 cup edamame, 130 calories / GF / DF
- Bellweather Farms plain sheep's milk yogurt, 140 calories / GF / DF
- Vermont Smoke and Cure Real Sticks (BBQ Flavor), 90 calories / GF / DF / Antibiotics and Sodium Nitrite free
- Paleovalley beef stick, 70 calories / GF
- Hard-boiled egg (free range), 60 calories / GF / DF
- Protein shake (pre-mixed in a to-go shaker bottle)

- Justin's almond butter squeeze packs (pre-portioned), 210 calories / GF
- Quaker rice cakes, 35 calories / GF (flavored rice cakes make great options, too)
- 1 tablespoon Smucker's sugar-free jam, 10 calories / GF

Natural Sweeteners that easily fit in a purse or portable cooler:

- Sweet Leaf or Now brand stevia (comes in small bottle with dropper and powder form)
- Monk fruit / lakanto dropper bottle
- Truvia sweetener packets

Ideas for Freezer Storage

When you can't make it to the grocery store or you didn't have a chance to do your meal prep, these store-bought freezer items are great for when you get home late and don't feel like cooking.

- Amy's frozen burritos (gluten and dairy free options)
- Frozen meals from Amy's, Applegate, or Kashi (or any brand you love, but watch the calories and any extreme sodium levels)
- Frozen bison or turkey patties
- Keep frozen loaves of your favorite whole grain or gluten-free bread
- Frozen berries (to make a quick smoothie)
- Frozen leftovers

Most of the portable snack items on this list, with a few exceptions, are foods that will keep in a cool spot for many months. I really encourage you to purchase a small, soft-sided cooler to keep in your car. Pack it full of healthy options so you always have snacks available to grab when you need them. I always keep meat sticks/beef jerky in my purse or travel bag in case I'm stuck somewhere without access to a solid, healthy meal. You learn through trial and error which snacks are the most satisfying and appealing to you.

If you crave things like chips or popcorn, take Ziplock bags and make portion-sized baggies to keep in your pantry. The same goes for crackers. You don't need to eliminate everything you love, but it's important to immediately store them in portioned baggies to prevent binging on open bags.

This is just a starting reference. The main idea is to plan ahead and keep plenty of stored healthy food so you always have good options to choose from and never go unprepared. Find the foods and snacks you love the most, because if you enjoy what you're eating, you are more likely to stick with your plan, make better choices, and feel better inside and out.

APPENDIX B
Sample Grocery List

Here are some options when stocking your pantry with healthy, fresh choices:

Proteins

- Chicken breast (hormone-free, free-range if possible)
- Tuna (albacore, water-packed)
- Eggs (cage-free, hormone-free if possible)
- Salmon (wild-caught when available)
- Turkey (extra lean, ground)
- Shrimp
- Bison (ground)

Nuts, Seeds, and Nut Butters

Raw is the best option for nuts and seeds. This way you minimize added oil and salt, but you can still get roasted versions if you're not ready to jump into the salt-free kind.

- Almonds
- Cashews
- Walnuts
- Pumpkin seeds

- Almond butter or peanut butter (pure nut butter, no added sugar or sweeteners)
- Tahini

Fruits

- All berries fresh or frozen (strawberries, blueberries, raspberries, blackberries)
- Bananas
- Apples
- Avocados
- Oranges
- Lemons & limes (to slice up for flavored water)
- Peaches
- Pears

Vegetables

It's a great time-saver to purchase vegetables pre-chopped or sliced. This is my list, but in reality, you can have almost any vegetable you like, except for corn and peas. Corn and peas should be eaten in measured amounts since they tend to be higher in calories than other vegetables.

- Broccoli
- Asparagus
- Cabbage
- Carrots
- Bell peppers
- Spinach
- Sweet potatoes

- Lettuce
- Squash (all varieties)
- Mushrooms

Sweeteners

- Honey
- Pure maple syrup
- Unsweetened applesauce
- Monk fruit (calorie-free, works well in baked goods)
- Stevia (calorie-free)
- Swerve (calorie-free, works well in baked goods)

Oils, Fats, and Sprays

- Olive oil (extra virgin)
- Spectrum coconut oil spray or olive oil spray (to coat cooking pans)
- Coconut oil
- Ghee

Pantry Items

- Balsamic vinegar
- Apple cider vinegar
- Celtic sea salt
- Herbamare
- All spices and herbs
- Marinara sauce (no added sugar)
- Coconut aminos (great to sauté with)

- Ketchup (sugar-free)
- Hot sauce (Cholula)
- Dijon mustard
- Salsa
- Herb teas & green teas
- Tamari (gluten-free, low-sodium)

APPENDIX C
Macro Reference Guide

(P=protein, C=carbohydrates, F=fat)

Protein	Serving	Calories	P	C	F
Chicken breast skinless, boneless	3 oz	128	23 g	0 g	2.7 g
Ground turkey 99% lean	4 oz	120	26 g	0 g	1.5 g
Ground beef 93% lean	4 oz	170	23g	0 g	8 g
Ground bison	4 oz	190	20 g	0 g	11 g
Salmon	4 oz	166	24.5 g	0 g	6.7 g
Shrimp	4 oz	100	21 g	0 g	1.5 g
Eggs, whole	1 large	74	6.2 g	0 g	4.9 g
Tuna water packed, albacore	4 oz	132	28 g	0 g	0.9 g
Greek yogurt plain, 0%	8 oz	130	22 g	11 g	0 g
Liquid egg whites	½ c.	75	5 g	1 g	0 g

Carbohydrates	Serving	Calories	P	C	F
Rolled oats uncooked	½ c.	150	6 g	27 g	2.5 g
White rice, cooked	1 c.	204	4.2 g	44 g	0.44 g
Sweet potato, diced	1 c.	110	2 g	26 g	0 g
Pasta, cooked, penne	1 c.	220	8 g	43 g	1.2 g
Ezekiel bread	1 slice	80	4 g	15 g	0.5 g
Sweet corn	½ c.	60	2 g	11 g	0.5 g
Banana	1 medium	105	1 g	27 g	0.3 g
Quinoa, cooked	1 c.	229	8 g	42 g	3.5 g

Fats	Serving	Calories	P	C	F
Avocado (fresh)	½ medium	130	1 g	1g	12g
Olive oil	1 tbs.	119	0 g	0 g	13.5 g
Coconut oil	1 tbs.	120	0 g	0 g	14 g
Butter	1 tbs.	102	0.1 g	0 g	11.5 g
Almond butter	1 tbs.	101	2.4 g	3 g	9.4 g

Fats	Serving	Calories	P	C	F
Walnuts	1 oz	185	4 g	4 g	18 g
Olives, Kalamata	5 whole	45	0 g	1 g	4.5 g
Parmesan cheese	1 tbs.	21	1.8 g	0.17 g	1.4 g
Sunflower seeds, ra)	¼ c.	170	7 g	6 g	15 g

APPENDIX D
Seasonal Produce Guide

As you increase the number of fresh fruits and vegetables in your diet, you'll soon discover that it can get a little pricey, especially if you shop for organics. There are ways of keeping costs down, however. One way is to only buy enough for each week to ensure that nothing goes bad. And then use it all before your next shopping trip.

Another great place to find better prices is at your local farmer's market. A lot of produce is priced better than what you might find at the grocery store, because they don't have the added costs of grocery store overhead (for example, importing produce from out of state and transportation).

If you shop for what's in season, you can cut costs, too. Seasonal produce is usually fresher, it tastes better, and it may last longer. So, use this seasonal produce guide for quick reference to reduce your costs at the store.

SPRING

apricots, artichokes, arugula, asparagus, chard, cherries, grapefruit, kiwis, leeks, lemons, lettuce, peas, radishes, spinach, strawberries, turnips

SUMMER

apples, apricots, avocados, bell peppers, blackberries, blueberries, cantaloupes, chard, corn, cucumbers, grapes, limes, mangoes, melons, nectarines, peaches

FALL

apples, arugula, beets, broccoli raabe, carrots, cauliflower, celery, cranberries, eggplant, figs, grapes, green beans, mushrooms, okra, peppers, sweet potatoes

WINTER

beets, broccoli, Brussels sprouts, cabbage, carrots, cauliflower, celery, clementines, kale, mandarins, onions, oranges, parsnips, pears, potatoes, winter squash

APPENDIX E
References

Part I: Introduction

Introduction to The Strategies, The Preparation

Aragon, A. (2022). *Flexible Dieting*. Las Vegas: Victory Belt Publishing Inc.

Brennan, D. (2021, May 05). *Differences Between BMR and RMR*. WebMD. https://www.webmd.com/fitness-exercise/difference-between-bmr-and-rmr

Chao, A.M., Quigley, K.M., & Wadden, T.A. (2021, January 4). Dietary interventions for obesity: clinical and mechanistic findings. *The Journal of Clinical Investigation*. https://doi.org/10.1172/jci140065

Part II: Nourishment Strategies – Food / Diet

Strategy 1 – Liquid Calories

Mayo Clinic Staff. (2023, January 18). *Counting Calories: Get Back to Weight Loss Basics*. Mayo Clinic. https://www.mayoclinic.org/healthy-lifestyle/weight-loss/in-depth/calories/art-20048065

The Sweet Danger of Sugar. (2022, January 6). Harvard Health Publishing. Retrieved Month Date, Year , from https://www.health.harvard.edu/heart-health/the-sweet-danger-of-sugar

Strategy 2 – The Breakfast Strategy

Duan, D., Pilla, S.J., Michalski, K., Laferrère, B., Clark, J.M., & Maruthur, N.M. (2022, February) Eating breakfast is associated with weight loss during an intensive lifestyle intervention for overweight/obesity. *The Obesity Society. 30*(2). 378-388. https://doi.org/10.1002/oby.23340

Hill, L. (2021, April 22). *Breakfast: Is it The Most Important Meal?* WebMD. https://www.webmd.com/food-recipes/breakfast-lose-weight

Strategy 3 – The Two-Hour Rule

Breus, M. (2019, June 02). *What Can Intermittent Fasting Do for Your Sleep?* Psychology Today. https://www.psychologytoday.com/us/blog/sleep-newzzz/201906/what-can-intermittent-fasting-do-your-sleep#:~:text=Some%20studies%20suggest%20that%20periodic%2C%20short-term%20fasting%20can,has%20shown%20that%20fasting%20may%20decrease%20REM%20sleep.

Strategy 4 – Fiber

Dietary Fiber: Essential for a Healthy Diet. (2022, November 04). Mayo Clinic. Retrieved Month Date, Year, from https://www.mayoclinic.org/healthy-lifestyle/nutrition-and-healthy-eating/in-depth/fiber/art-20043983

Strategy 5 – The Vegetable Edge

Health Benefits of Vegetables. (2022, September 21). WebMD. Retrieved Month Date, Year, from https://www.webmd.com/diet/health-benefits-vegetables

Strategy 6 – Protein Strategies

Aragon, A. (2022). *Flexible Dieting.* Las Vegas: Victory Belt Publishing Inc.

Dieter, B. (2022). *Protein and Weight Loss: How Much Protein Do You Need to Eat Per Day?* NASM. https://blog.nasm.org/nutrition/how-much-protein-should-you-eat-per-day-for-weight-loss

Strategy 8 – Gut Health: Eliminating What Doesn't Work

Understanding Gut Health: Signs of an Unhealthy Gut and What to Do About It. (2022, June 01). Healthline. Retrieved Month Date, Year, from https://www.healthline.com/health/gut-health#gut-microbiome

Strategy 10 – Estrogens and Obesogens

Frye, C.A., Bo, E., Calamandrei, G., Calzà, L., Dessì-Fulgheri, F., Fernández, M., Fusani, L., Kah, O., Kajta, M., Le Page, Y., Patisaul, H.B., Venerosi, A., Wojtowicz, A.K., & Panzica, G.C. Endocrine disrupters: a review of some sources, effects, and mechanisms of actions on behaviour and neuroendocrine systems. *Journal of Neuroendocrinology. 24*(1). 144-159. https://doi.org/10.1111/j.1365-2826.2011.02229.x

Holtcamp, W. (2012, February). Obesogens: An Environmental *Link to Obesity.* Environmental Health Perspectives. https://ehp.niehs.nih.gov/doi/10.1289/ehp.120-a62

Part III: Movement, Rest and Progress Strategies

Strategy 12 – Sleep

Mann, D. (2013, April 30). *Sleep and Weight Gain: Will better sleep help you avoid extra pounds?* WebMD. https://www.webmd.com/sleep-disorders/features/lack-of-sleep-weight-gain

Schmid, S.M., Hallschmid, M., Jauch-Chara, K., Born, J., & Schultes, B. (2008). A single night of sleep deprivation increases ghrelin levels and feelings of hunger in normal-weight healthy men. *Journal of Sleep Research. 17*(3). 331-334. https://doi.org/10.1111/j.1365-2869.2008.00662.x

Strategy 13 – The NEAT Strategy

Comana, F. (2022). *Non-Exercise Activity Thermogenesis: A NEAT Approach to Weight Loss.* NASM. https://blog.nasm.org/exercise-programming/neat-approach-weight-loss

Use the NEAT Factor (nonexercised activity thermogenesis) to Burn Calories. (2015, January 28). Harvard Health Publishing. Retrieved Month Date, Year, from https://www.health.harvard.edu/diet-and-weight-loss/use-the-neat-factor-nonexercise-activity-thermogenesis-to-burn-calories

Strategy 14 – Exercise

Exercise: 7 Benefits of Regular Activity. (2021, October 08). Mayo Clinic. Retrieved Month Date, Year, from https://www.mayoclinic.org/healthy-lifestyle/fitness/in-depth/exercise/art-20048389#:~:text=Exercise%3A%207%20benefits%20of%20regular%20physical%20activity%201,Need%20an%20emotional%20lift%3F%20...%20More%20items...%20

Strategy 15 – Weighing Progress

Armitage, H. (2021, February 24). *Digital Health Tracking Tools help Individuals Lose Weight, study finds.* Stanford Medicine. https://med.stanford.edu/news/all-news/2021/02/digital-health-tracking-tools-help-individuals-lose-weight-study-finds.html

Bjarnadottir, A. (2017, January 03). *How Often Should I Weigh Myself?* Healthline. https://www.healthline.com/health/diet-and-weight-loss/how-often-should-i-weigh-myself

Strategy 16 – Macros, Prepping and Tracking

Armitage, H. (2021, February 24). *Digital Health Tracking Tools help Individuals Lose Weight, study finds.* Stanford Medicine. https://med.stanford.edu/news/all-news/2021/02/digital-health-tracking-tools-help-individuals-lose-weight-study-finds.html

Duke University. (2019, February 28). *Tracking food leads to losing pounds: Those who tracked food and weight lost pounds in new study. ScienceDaily.* www.sciencedaily.com/releases/2019/02/190228154839.htm

Part IV: Mindset Strategies

Strategy 17 – Visualizing Your Success

Adams, A.J. (2009, December 03). *Seeing is Believing: The power of visualization.* Psychology Today. https://www.psychologytoday.com/us/blog/flourish/200912/seeing-is-believing-the-power-visualization#:~:text=Brain%20studies%20now%20reveal%20that%20thoughts%20produce%20the,is%20getting%20trained%20for-%20actual%20performance%20during%20visualization.

Brenner, A. (2016, June 25). *The Benefits of Creative Visualization*. Psychology Today. https://www.psychologytoday.com/us/blog/in-flux/201606/the-benefits-creative-visualization

Strategy 18 – Feeding Your Mind

Davey, G. (2020, September 21). The Psychological Impact of Negative News: Negative news can significantly affect our mental health. Psychology Today. https://www.psychologytoday.com/us/blog/why-we-worry/202009/the-psychological-impact-negative-news

Strategy 20 – The Missing Element

Social Support: A Necessity for Weight Loss. (2023). Mayo Clinic. Retrieved Month Date, Year, from https://diet.mayoclinic.org/us/blog/2021/social-support-a-necessity-for-weight-loss/

Conclusion

Huberman, A. (2024). *David Goggins: How to Build Immense Inner Strength*. Wisdom in a Nutshell.

Acknowledgements

In publishing my first book, I have become aware of the tremendous amount of work required and, subsequently, the value of support, encouragement, and skilled feedback. There are many people to thank, and I will undoubtedly miss a few. I especially want to give thanks to Stacy Dymalski for her feedback and suggestions. Callie Miller's skillful copy editing and refining touches are most appreciated. I want to thank Michelle Reyner of Cosmic Design and Katie Mullaly of Surrogate Press for pulling it all together with beautiful design and guidance. Most of all, I want to thank Jim for believing in me and for your unrelenting encouragement, despite my doubts, to follow through in pursuing my passion for sharing my hard-earned knowledge.

About the Author

Cynthia began her health and fitness journey early in life as an overweight child struggling to find a weight loss solution in the late seventies when there was no internet and very few reliable sources of information. Her endeavors were all trial and error and almost entirely unsuccessful. Her unyielding determination finally resulted in the weight loss success she had been yearning for, though not without utilizing some unhealthy tactics.

Hoping to find the safest, most sustainable solutions, her efforts eventually led to a strong desire to learn more, and she enrolled at The University of Rhode Island and earned a bachelor's degree in Dietetics and Nutrition after which she moved to Florida and became a personal trainer. Working with clients for several years further fueled her desire for more education and the need to make a more direct impact on people's lives.

This aspiration to learn more led to a master's degree as well as an additional Bachelor of Science in nursing and she has been a Registered Nurse since 2010, with direct patient care in areas such as inpatient and emergency medicine.

For over thirty years Cynthia has continued to follow her passion for fitness and health with continuing education on the latest peer-reviewed data available on topics related to nutrition and exercise. This pursuit has led to the development of the strategies outlined in this book which she hopes can help others achieve their own success in developing and maintaining lifelong health.

www.ingramcontent.com/pod-product-compliance
Lightning Source LLC
Chambersburg PA
CBHW060233030426
42335CB00014B/1443
* 9 7 8 1 9 4 7 4 5 9 9 9 1 *